CAREERS IN HEALTH

CAREERS IN HEALTH

THE PROFESSIONALS GIVE YOU THE INSIDE PICTURE

ABOUT THEIR JOBS

Barbara Zimmermann / David B. Smith

BEACON PRESS : BOSTON

Copyright © 1978 by Barbara Zimmermann and David B. Smith
Beacon Press books are published under the auspices
of the Unitarian Universalist Association
Published simultaneously in Canada by
Fitzhenry & Whiteside Limited, Toronto
Published simultaneously in hardcover and paperback editions
All rights reserved
Printed in the United States of America

(paperback)   9   8   7   6   5   4   3   2   1
(hardcover)   9   8   7   6   5   4   3   2   1

Library of Congress Cataloging in Publication Data

Zimmermann, Barbara, 1945–
    Careers in health.

    1. Medicine—Vocational guidance.   2. Allied
health personnel—Vocational guidance.   I. Smith,
David Barton, joint author.   II. Title.
R690.Z55   610.69′5   78–53788
ISBN 0–8070–2578–X
ISBN 0–8070–2579–8 pbk.

For Henry, sine qua non

ACKNOWLEDGMENTS

This book could not have been written without the kind cooperation of the health workers whose stories are presented. We are most grateful to them for sharing their work days and their thoughts. We hope we have adequately described the impressive commitment these people have made to their work.

On the Iowa side, a special thanks goes to Varena Wade for her typing services and her encouragement during the final preparations.

From the Philadelphia side, a number of people, in addition to those who served as subjects for chapters, deserve thanks. The cheerful assistance given by Frances French, Karen Philiczak, Cindy Jones and Gwendolyn Howard in typing final drafts of the manuscript under very tight deadlines was gratefully appreciated. Colleagues in the Department of Health Administration at Temple University, Mike Dolfman, Chuck Hall, and Harry Karpeles, provided assistance in obtaining local contacts and much encouragement. Miriam Adler, and avid reader of young adult mystery stories, and Nancy Woollcott Smith, a writer of them, read most of the chapters and gave us a number of useful suggestions. Thanks are also due former colleague William Barker of the Department of Preventive and Community Medicine at the University of Rochester who gave encouragement to the project in its early stages and supplied some ideas for positions to be included in one of the appendices. William Allen and Ann Garland of the Department of Health of the City of Philadelphia were kind enough to review the material on related positions for the preventive health section and gave a number of useful suggestions. Finally, I would like to thank my wife, Adelheid Sannwald, for her even-tempered patience and gentle support in the most discouraging stages of this effort.

INTRODUCTION

A young person planning a career today views a complicated scene. Modern technology has exploded a limited occupational picture into a jungle of well over 20,000 official job titles. This book is written for people trying to approach that jungle. It is about health occupations, an area that has been changed perhaps more than any by modern technology. Professional health care today includes a range of workers, medications and equipment not dreamed of even thirty years ago. The number of people employed in the health sector has grown to five million and will continue to grow.

Health occupations offer a tremendous variety of career possibilities. The modern health system has new roles for doctors and nurses, as well as new paramedical, technical and support careers. These occupations do not all require years of education. They do not all require an interest in science, or a strong stomach or even a special ability with people. They do require a commitment to doing a job well. Whether the task is listening to a heart beat, or looking at a blood smear through a microscope, it has ultimately to do with the welfare of a fellow human being.

The best way to learn about health occupations would be to spend time with people on the job, in hospitals, clinics, doctors' offices and public health departments where the work of health care is largely done. You could see for yourself what the different jobs involve, what seems boring, exciting, or disgusting. You could ask the workers how they feel about their work.

In the work life portraits that follow, we have tried to convey the experience of spending time on the job with health care workers. The workers you will read about are real people. The days we have tried to capture are real, and the feelings about work and health care expressed are those of the workers. To cover questions you cannot ask, we have provided a job summary at the end of each chapter, with salary expectations, duties, and a list of training programs and addresses to write to for more information.

The workers are divided into five sections. The section called "The New Practitioners" will introduce you to a new group of workers who are now trained to do work that was once reserved for nurses and doctors. The second section is called "New Jobs for Old Practitioners." Here you will meet people in the more traditional medical occupations whose roles have changed in modern medicine. "Technicians and Therapists" will touch on some of the many new diagnostic and therapeutic workers who are part of the medical team. "The Organizers" will focus on the wide range of managers and coordinators who keep the system going. "Protectors of Health" presents some of the workers in the growing area of public health and preventive medicine. At the end of each section we have supplied a brief catalogue of "Related Occupations."

The final chapter of the book will provide a view of the health-care system, how it works, what its future may be, and will also give you some direction in finding your place in it.

The picture you get of the health-care system will not be a romantic one. We feel you need more than a pep talk, a list of qualifications and a salary schedule to approach a career decision. You need to listen to people on the front line and to mentally try on their shoes.

The romantic image of health care presented in some literature cannot adequately sustain workers through what is often difficult, discouraging and even thankless work. But if you believe in doing a job well, and in sometimes quiet and unheralded magic, we hope that you find something of interest in the chapters that follow.

new practitioners

New practitioners occupy the new positions in the health field. They have some of the same autonomy in providing patient care that, until recently, was only enjoyed by physicians. They are also filling an important gap in the health-care system by providing care to people who weren't able to get it before. The physician's assistant whom you will meet in the first chapter is one of a new group of practitioners who are making it possible for people in isolated and underdoctored areas to get primary care. The home health aide in chapter 2 is helping to make home care a reality. The emergency medical technician in chapter 3 is helping to extend the lifesaving capability of hospitals and physicians throughout communities.

Although their numbers are still quite small, positions of this kind are growing more rapidly than any others in the health sector. There is a widespread public acceptance of physician's assistants. The public likes to see a practitioner quickly and have more time with him or her to get their questions answered. Evaluations have shown that physician's assistants provide as good or better quality of care, within their restricted area of competence, as their supervising physicians. They haven't won full acceptance by the medical profession yet, however. Some physicians worry about the malpractice problems that might result from employing them. There are also some physicians who have a strong reluctance to delegate patient care responsibilities.

New public support of home health and emergency medical services are producing an increasing need for people in these areas. If given a choice, most people who are ill would probably rather stay home than go to a nursing home or hospital. The development of home care programs makes that choice possible. Home health aides are an important part of such programs. They have a far greater degree of autonomy in such work than the nurse's aides, who have a similar amount of training but work in hospitals or nursing homes.

Emergency medical technicians are perhaps the most recent of the new practitioners. Recent advances in medical technology have made it possible to bring lifesaving equipment out of the hospital and to the side of the patient. Emergency medical technicians serve as the key link in systems that are developing across the country to save lives in medical emergencies.

1.

PHYSICIAN'S ASSISTANT

The somber grey of the long corridor is broken by bright directional arrows hung at intervals from the ceiling. At one end of the corridor, a yellow arrow with white letters reads Primary Care. Toward the middle, a red arrow marks Surgery and at the other end, a blue arrow points left to General Medicine. Patients coming to this large Veterans Administration Hospital go to one of these three areas.

Janet Thompson works in the General Medicine Clinic, one of two physician's assistants hired in this clinic a year and a half ago. "Physician's assistant" (PA) is a relatively new title, although doctors have always assigned work to aides. What is new is the development of formal programs to train people for tasks previously requiring a doctor. The return of Vietnam medical corpsmen, men with great medical experience but no license to use it off the battlefield, was a factor in starting the first physician's assistant training program.

Janet's office is just past the General Medicine waiting room, a carpeted break in the grey tile bordered by the waist-high planters. Unlike most office greenery, there are real plants in the boxes, but they have been all but smothered by cigarette butts and candy bar wrappers.

Janet is twenty-five years old. She is big but gives the impression of energy and strength, rather than heaviness. There is a steady, insistent gaze from her eyes. Even sitting quietly at her desk she seems energetic. She is wearing a long white lab coat with her name and title, Physician's Assistant, pinned to it. Underneath the coat is a turtleneck sweater and a pair of corduroy pants.

She is a graduate of the Duke University physician's assistant program. She shares her office with another physician's assistant, John Murphy, also a Duke graduate.

Janet and John were the first physician's assistants to be hired at this VA Hospital. They have a permanent staff doctor as their director, but their immediate supervisor is the resident physician doing his month-long rotation in the General Medicine clinic.

"This is a very different situation than when a PA works for a single doctor," Janet says. "It means the degree of responsibility we are given varies from month to month. Sometimes we have a resident who checks us constantly. Maybe because we make a mistake in the beginning, or maybe she or he just doesn't trust the idea of physician's assistants. The next month we may be more independent. It's up to the resident."

"Our training was really thorough," Janet says. "One year of classroom work, roughly what the medical students take, and a year of rotations. I wouldn't know how to draw the line between what we're trained to do and what a doctor is trained to do. We don't have as many rotations. Like, I've never been on a burn unit or in a delivery room. But some PAs have. I guess the difference would be in degree. The doctors have more experience, more classroom training right along the line. That's why we're under a doctor's supervision. Although sometimes . . ." Janet reaches for a cigarette and lights it slowly. "Well, sometimes I've found myself knowing more or having more skill than a particular doctor I'm working with. It was a surprise to me. There's just no clear division."

Janet's day begins around eight-thirty in the morning. She stops first at the reception and appointment desk to look over her morning schedule.

"Our patients come from three sources," Janet says as she bends over the large sheets on the calendar. "We see new patients, returns and sometimes referrals from other parts of the hospital." She goes to the patient chart file and pulls out the records for the return patients she will be seeing that day.

"Oh no, not this guy!" she grimaces as she walks across the hall to her office and drops the records down on a large desk. John is already at his desk, writing up patient records from the previous day. There is an examining table in the room, with a blood pressure gauge and a supply table for use on busy days.

Today is not a busy day. It is the Friday before Christmas and it has snowed heavily during the night, making highway travel difficult. Because it is connected with a university hospital, this VA has a particularly good reputation. It is not unusual for patients to come two or three hundred miles, often from other states, just for a yearly checkup. The medical care, including any drugs prescribed, is free to veterans. Patients with high incomes are supposed to pay something, but there is little checking.

"Unless the person's name was Rockefeller or something, there would not be any outside check," Janet says. "I doubt there is much cheating. For anyone with money, the VA is a comedown, like welfare or something." She glances quickly through the files on her desk from the day before and begins writing up unfinished records.

"John, I've got that nut this morning. You know, the one that was here a couple of weeks ago? He was drunk and threatened to sue the hospital for something or other. Where's Fred?"

"He's in the staff lounge. The secretaries brought cookies because it's his last day of rotation."

"No, I'm here." Dr. Fred Hansen, the current resident on duty, walks into the office, a styrofoam cup of coffee in one hand and a brownie in the other. He is a tall, slender person with a wide blond mustache. His white pants and jacket are floppy on him, but too short at the wrists and ankles.

"Hi, Fred." Janet motions him to the chart on her desk. "Remember this guy?" Fred looks at the chart briefly and smiles. "Well, all the tests for ulcers were negative, but if he still has pain, I think I'll start him on the ulcer regime anyway. The guy's life is a mess. I think it would be a good approach for him."

"That sounds fine. How about the tranquilizers?"

"I'll give him a refill on the Valium."

"OK. Call me if he gives you any trouble."

"I will. Where are you going after Christmas?" Janet asks.

"Cardiology. You should try these brownies. They're great."

"No thanks. If I gain any more weight I'll end up as your patient over there."

Janet returns to the charts on her desk. The first hour and a half in the morning is usually spent catching up on paper work. Then she picks up a chart and goes out to the waiting room.

"Frank Pierson?" she calls. The waiting room is full now, mostly with older men. The man who steps forward is young. "Hi Frank,"

Janet smiles. "Let's go down the hall here." Frank is short and wiry. He wears a suede jacket with the collar up and a 1950s "greaser" hair style. He keeps his hands in his pockets as he walks. In the examining room he sits at a corner table with Janet. He keeps his hands in his lap and his thumbs twirl constantly. He is only twenty-one, but his face is lined with strain.

"How are things going, Frank?"

"Oh, not real good, I guess."

"Well, let's start with the stomach pains. Have you been taking the tranquilizers?"

"Yeah, they help a little. I don't know. Still quite a bit of pain at night."

"I told you when you were here last that we didn't find any concrete signs of an ulcer, but that doesn't mean you don't have the beginnings of one. I think we'll start you on an ulcer regime. It will be better for your body and nerves, ulcer or not." Janet uses her hands vigorously as she speaks, but her voice is slow and gentle.

"Yeah, I'm so nervous. Like today, driving to the hospital. I almost freaked out. The roads weren't bad or anything but I was just nervous the whole time."

"How much are you smoking?"

"Oh, pack, pack and a half."

"The first thing on the ulcer regime is cutting out the cigarettes and booze."

"Oh God." He laughs nervously, and pushes his hands through his hair.

"I know it's not easy, believe me. I smoke myself. But as long as you keep up the smoking and drinking, you're going to have the pain. You think the smoking helps when you're nervous, but it's really aggravating things. Whatever you can cut out will help."

"It's just with all the problems, I'm so tense. I come home from work . . . you see, the drinking just seems to calm me down and I smoke when I drink."

"And then the pain starts in the evening, right?"

"Yeah."

"Is there anyone you could talk things out with? I mean, instead of using alcohol. How about your wife?"

"Naw, I can't talk to her at all."

"Well, do you have a friend?"

"Yeah, but he drinks." They both laugh.

"How is your baby son doing?"

"Not so good. He's back in the hospital again. I don't know what they're doing. They're running some kind of sweat test on him. I don't know. The last time he was in it ran up something like seven hundred dollars. And then they wanted to fire me from the morgue for drinking."

"You've got to keep yourself together. Your baby is sick, and things are really down for you. Taking care of your *own* body is important for him too. I'm not going to have you make another appointment. Just come in if you feel like you need more help. If you're going to be in the area, give a call and I'll see you. We'll work on adjusting your diet again. If that doesn't work, we'll try some other approach. But give this a whirl first." Janet stands up and they both walk back toward the waiting room.

"If you'll just wait here a minute, I'll get Dr. Hansen to co-sign this prescription for you."

Fred is back in the lounge by the coffee machine and Janet hands the prescription to him.

"No troubles?" he asks, as he writes.

"No. He's pretty calm today. Nothing much to offer him. At least he was friendly."

She goes back to Frank, who is waiting in the hall.

"You know where to get this filled? OK. Good luck. Now stop in again if you feel you need more help."

Janet goes back to her desk and makes some notes on Frank's record.

"I'm afraid he's one who will be back in a few years with liver problems and the whole works. There's so little you can do with someone like that." Janet broods and lights a cigarette.

"If I ever thought of this job in terms of helping people, I'd go nuts. I used to believe in helping people. But it was a terrible ego trip for me. I wanted people to like me. I'd help them so they would like me. If I couldn't help them, I figured they wouldn't like me. I ended up not liking anyone I couldn't help. It was ridiculous."

Janet's next patient is returning for a six-week check. He is thirty-six, neatly dressed and has a beard that, even freshly shaven, gives a shadowy look to his face. His problem had been tension headaches and weakness in a leg that was scarred. Janet checks him on the exercises she prescribed and finds the leg stronger.

"I don't think I'll need to see you again unless you notice some change in the leg," Janet says.

"Oh, by the way," he says as he stands to leave. "I was wondering if I might be able to get compensation for the leg . . ."

"Oh gee, I couldn't tell you," Janet answers. "You'd have to go to the compensation and pension office for that. Take a left on the main corridor. There's a big glass window at the end with an orange sign over it."

"Well . . . thanks."

"Nice to see you doing so well." Janet turns and heads back toward her office. "That does irk me," she mutters. John has left a cup of coffee for her on the desk and she sits with it and makes some notes. "It makes you a little suspicious. Around here, everyone wants compensation for something. It's so typical for people to go on and on about a complaint, and they'll ask you at the last minute, sort of casually, about compensation. Not that he was only after that. But it can make you very cynical, guessing about half-sick people, the whiners, the crocks, when there are so many really sick people around. I feel bad, but I get annoyed too. I never thought I would resent any of the financial aspects of patient care. I just can't help thinking . . . well, there's a patient I'll be seeing later this morning, who lost his leg in a mine explosion in Vietnam. He doesn't complain, he doesn't ask for special treatment. I'm being unfair. It's something you have to resist all the time, just losing respect for people a bit. The crocks need help too. I know that in my head. And in some ways it's what I like about being a physician's assistant. The MDs, they're always pressed. We have time to listen. These crocky complaints can be part of serious problems. A busy physician may not take time to follow them all up. Also, spending time going over details, like an ulcer regime, or the use of medications, is PA work. Most doctors don't take time to explain why a particular drug or diet works. We get a lot of arthritics here. It's terribly important that they understand aspirin therapy . . . the dosages, how to tell if they have overdosed, how to tell if they need a substitute aspirin. Most arthritics have never heard any details on this therapy. We can do a lot of education and preventive medicine that is neglected by physicians. It's satisfying to feel you are being thorough, at least most of the time.

"People ask me, well, you've had two years of training, why didn't you go the extra time and become a doctor? You can't help thinking about that, especially once you start working and realize how closely your functions are related to those of a physician. One problem would be getting into medical school, of course. Even with my BA, I would have to go back and take at least a year of organic chemistry and physics. And then what? I'd have no guarantee of getting into medical school. More than that, though, is the lifestyle. The way things are now, to be a physician, medicine has to be your whole life. I want a personal life too. Maybe children, maybe a home in the country with my husband. I want time for friends and for hobbies. Being a physician's assistant I am involved in medicine, in intensive diagnostic work, in interesting patient contact, not just a routine, and yet I don't have to sacrifice other fulfillments. As far as being independent, it just depends on the job. Some PAs are independent, that is, physically removed from the physician. You do get more independent as you gain experience. The jobs vary tremendously. Our job placement office kept a file of physicians who had asked about getting a PA. They were asked to describe their needs, the average number of hours they put in, stuff like that. The main thing the doctors had in common was that hardly any of them put in less than seventy or eighty hours a week. I want to avoid that kind of situation."

Janet finishes her coffee and a cigarette and reaches for another patient chart. "Mr. Beam has been waiting a while. I guess I'd better get to him. He was in two weeks ago, pains in his chest, under his rib cage. We found a hiatal hernia and got him on a hernia regime. He's coming back for a follow-up."

Mr. Beam is a man in his fifties. He is overweight, a problem that has settled mostly in his waistline and given him an older appearance. He has grey thinning hair and rather thick features. He is wearing a grey work uniform. He is very short of breath. Even sitting in the examining room he is panting.

"How are the chest pains, Mr. Beam?"

"Much better. I've been sleeping slanted, the way you told me, and the diet and everything. I've been sleeping better at night." His voice is raspy and broken.

"That's great. I was pretty sure that would help."

"I was wondering if you'd ... well, I've got this knee that has been giving me pain. I was wondering if you'd look at that. And also, my tummy. It seems awfully big and hard. I wonder if that's normal."

"How long has the knee been bothering you?"

"Oh, couple of weeks. I got laid off work at the plant. I've helped some guys move furniture. Heavier work than I'm used to."

"Mmmmm. Does it bother you all the time?"

"Mostly just when I go to stand up after sitting. Then I feel a sharp pain. The rest of the time, I don't notice it much."

"On the stomach, have you gained weight recently?"

"Well, some, yes. Since I've been off work. Maybe eight pounds."

"But the area feels different than before?"

"Yes, it's kind of hard."

"No pain?"

"Not really, no."

"OK, Mr. Beam, I want you to get undressed to your underwear and I'll take a look at both the knee and the stomach."

Janet makes some notes on her pad while Mr. Beam undresses and climbs on the examining table. His skin is pale and he has three large blue and red tattoos on one arm. The stomach he complained of looks smooth and tight bulging over the elastic on his underpants.

"OK, Mr. Beam, just sit with your legs over the side of the table. That's it." Janet steps back first to look at the knees together. Then she feels each one separately with her hand. "Yes, there is a little heat. Not much at all, and no redness." With fingers stretched outward, she moves her hands gently around the area of the kneecap on each leg. "Well, there is some fluid in that knee, but not much. We'll have you get an X ray just to make sure, but I suspect it's a minor strain. Now, let's have you lie down on your back." Janet reaches for the stethoscope in her coat pocket. "OK, now this is going to be a little cold. Just breathe normally for me, Mr. Beam. That's it." She moves the stethoscope slowly around the chest area. "Now I'm going to palpate your stomach area to check for any fluid build-up. My hands may be a little cold." She moves her hands, fingers stretched out, in circles around the enlarged stomach. Mr. Beam twitches.

"That tickles," he laughs hoarsely.

While Mr. Beam gets dressed, Janet writes out an X-ray order on a special prescription pad.

"I'm going to send you down to X ray," Janet says. "When you come back I'm going to have Dr. Hansen look at you, too."

Fred is in the PA's office, talking with John about a football game.

"Fred," Janet interrupts them. "Mr. Beam is going to X ray now. When he's done, would you look at him? There might be some fluid build-up in the abdomen. I couldn't tell. He has some beautiful tattoos."

"Dirty?"

"No, one was MOM. Faded though. Oh, I'd better call the lab. Mike Stanton was going there for blood tests before he came here." She picks up the white phone on her desk and dials a two-digit number.

"Yes, Janet Thompson in meds. Do you have a test back on Mike Stanton? Good. I'll be right down."

"Mike came in two weeks ago," Janet explains as she walks down the hall to the lab. "He's the Vietnam veteran who lost a leg. But he came in with fever and chills, vomiting, diarrhea. His blood tests showed this high elevation of a particular white cell. There are certain illnesses, jungle fever kinds of things, that you might look for in someone coming back from Vietnam, but nothing seemed to explain it. So we told him to come back in two weeks for some more blood tests."

Back in the office she hands Dr. Hansen the short white laboratory report.

"Weird, Fred, look. That eosinophil count is still ten times normal. Would you see him with me now?"

"Sure, let's go down to my office."

Mike is a hospital favorite. When he came back from Vietnam, his rehabilitation work was done at this VA and he is comfortable here. He is a big, handsome young man, with dark hair and eyes, and a gentle, awkward smile. His leg was amputated just below the knee. In his blue jeans and tall suede boots, there is nothing unusual about his appearance except for a slight limp and a thickness around the knee where the artificial limb is attached. Both Janet and Fred sit down with him in Fred's office.

"How are you feeling, Mike?" Fred asks.

"Fine. No fever. All the symptoms are gone. It was like I just had the flu or something."

"The tests show the white cell count is still quite high so it leaves us with a bit of a mystery. It's good that you're feeling better."

"Did you check with your family doctor about members of your family with the same elevation?" Janet asks.

"Yup. There wasn't anything. The doctor had pretty complete records too. Nothing."

"OK. Let me give you a going over on the examining table. Just take off your shirt and sit up there," Fred instructs.

Fred gives Mike a brief physical. Janet watches and records heart rate and other findings as Fred goes along.

"Everything seems fine," Fred says as Mike gets his shirt back on. "That leaves us in an awkward position. You seem healthy, and there may be nothing wrong. But that elevation is quite abnormal and we will definitely want to keep an eye on it. That means more blood tests, say every two weeks. I know it's a bit of a drive but it is important. In the meantime, if you have any flare-ups, diarrhea, fevers, anything unusual at all, we'll see you right away."

On their way back to the PA's office, Janet and Fred pick up their lunches from a small icebox in the office. Janet's is just a carton of yogurt.

"I've checked on everything," Fred says as he lifts himself onto the office examining table. "I looked up all the weird tropical diseases. I asked Dr. Farley too, and he said just to watch it. That's all we can do."

"He's such a nice fellow," Janet says. The phone rings. It is an orderly in the hospital who wants to talk to Janet about the physician's assistant program.

"It's really nice that people are learning about the program," she says after making arrangements to meet the caller after Christmas. "I mean, it was such an accident for me. There I was, four years of college and an English degree, no idea what I wanted to do. So I went to Boston to get a job and the only thing I could do was type. I went to work at a hospital because, for some reason, typing for a hospital seemed more relevant than typing for an insurance agent. Just being around a hospital you hear a lot, and I finally heard about the PA program. All those As in English, the BA, didn't mean a thing. I applied and was rejected . . . smacko! But I really was hooked, and for the first time in my life I got aggressive. I called the head of admissions and I said, 'Look, I want to know why I was rejected because I'm going to apply again.' He got my records and said, 'You don't have any experience with patient care.'

I said, 'How am I going to get experience? All I can do is type and write essays on Shakespeare.' He said, 'Come down and I'll find a job for you.' I was lucky. I went to North Carolina and worked on a surgery ward for a year. I was sort of a nurse's aide's aide. That's all they want. Orderly, bedpan supervisor . . . anything, just to make sure you can handle the patient contact. I think it's good. You get over the initial awful experiences before you start studying seriously." Janet scrapes the bottom of her yogurt carton thoughtfully with a plastic spoon.

"I think you remember those first experiences forever. In the surgery ward I worked on, they put the sickest patients, the ones who were dying, nearest the nursing station. On my first day of work I got my uniform on, and started padding along behind this nurse I was assigned to. We came to the room by the nursing station. I already had been told there was a dying man there. I walked in with the nurse.

"I don't know what I expected. He was dying of throat cancer, a youngish guy, maybe thirty-five, a high-school teacher. He had a tracheotomy, a hole in his neck so he could breathe because the growth had cut off his wind. The smell was terrible. But the thing that got to me was—he was just lying there. He knew he was dying and I expected him to be raging against death, or shouting 'I'm dying, I'm dying,' but he was just lying there, watching.

"Well, the nurse did something or other and was moving around and I was standing there. What I did was pass out. I knew I couldn't pass out in front of the patient but I just lost consciousness. I managed to follow the nurse out of the room into the hall and I called to her. I think I said 'Hey you,' because I forgot her name. I couldn't see anything. I walked across the corridor and flat into a wall. After that I don't know what happened.

"But the next time I went into his room, I was ready. It isn't deliberate, but you have this built-in reaction—his death is my death—and when that sank in I just went blank. Total denial.

"I've never worked in a really gory setting, like emergency or burns. I did work in surgery for a while. I liked that a lot although I got so I was falling asleep during long operations. The doc I was working with would nudge me and say 'Fascinating, eh Janet?' Basically, I like human bodies."

Janet goes on. "Even someone like Mr. Beam. God knows he's not attractive, blotchy dry skin. But I don't mind touching him.

What bothers me most is smells. Last week I had an alcoholic, an old guy. He hadn't bathed for years, I'm sure. God, it was incredible. I was in the middle of listening to his heart and I had to walk out of the room to keep from puking."

"It seems like everyone has one thing that really gets to them," Fred says. "For me, it's bloody stools. I'd walk through fire to avoid a bloody bedpan."

"It's vomit for me," John adds cheerfully. "I used to work in a recovery room. Everyone throwing up from the anesthetics. Piles and piles . . ."

"My lunch, John, my lunch," Janet pleads. She picks up the phone and dials out. "Janet Thompson in meds. Do you have an X ray done on Mr. Beam? He was just up a bit ago. Thanks, I'll hold . . . No? OK, we'll come up and find it." She hangs up the phone. "Fred, want to come up and find that X ray? It must be in the wrong slot or something. You're better at sniffing out X rays than I am."

They take an elevator to the X-ray room. In one corner there is a floor-to-ceiling alphabetized file, but Mr. Beam's X rays aren't under B. Instead, Fred finds them in a wire basket behind the file.

Fred clips the new X ray to a lighted viewing panel and Janet places the earlier one next to it.

"What a classic hiatal hernia," Fred breathes. "That's perfect. Well, the heart seems the same, no enlargement to speak of. This could be fluid here, but not much. Not enough to cause any tension in the area. Shall we look at the knee?"

"Nuts, it's not here," says Janet, checking the envelope again.

"Are you sure you wrote it down?"

"Yeah, look. It's right here. Will I have to send him up again?"

"We'll see. Probably a good idea."

Passing the waiting room in General Medicine, Janet calls to Mr. Beam. "Mr. Beam, this is Dr. Hansen. He's going to examine you and check your knee and stomach since he didn't see you last time."

"That's OK." Mr. Beam follows Janet down to an examining room and sits in a chair near Fred.

"Mr. Beam," Fred begins. "The stomach and the knee have just been bothering you recently, is that right?"

"Yes. Well, since I've been laid off work. We're going to Texas for Christmas and if I can find work there, we'll stay. I kind of wanted to get it checked before we left."

"I see. Well, I'd like you to take off everything but your underpants now, if you would, and sit up on the examining table." Fred gives Mr. Beam a routine physical. After checking everything out, he gives Mr. Beam a refill of the medication for his hernia symptoms and instructs him to lose weight. Mr. Beam leaves to go to the pharmacy and Janet returns to her office.

"Doesn't look like we're getting any new patients," Janet says, glancing at her watch. "Usually John and I will give the physicals before the resident is called in at all. I thought I would have problems giving physicals here, since the patients are mostly older, and almost all men. My first day I said, 'Now, Mr. so-and-so, I'm going to give you a rectal exam,' and the guy said 'Oh no you're not!' and I said, 'Yes I *am*!' and I did. I guess there was something unconfident about the way I said it the first time. I haven't had any trouble since. If you're relaxed and confident about what you're doing, there aren't many men who will complain."

A typical day for Janet usually includes three or four return patients in the morning, and then four or five new patients in the afternoon. Because of the snow and the upcoming holiday, she spends the afternoon catching up on paper work.

A PA student who has been doing a rotation in one of the wards upstairs stops to say good-bye, as does a secretary leaving for a Florida vacation. People begin to leave the clinic early since the snow is falling heavily and the highway report predicts hazardous driving.

"We have some dull days," Janet sighs. "When you start in medicine, you think the high points of your work are going to be connected with particular people you've helped, or dramatic situations, accidents, bizarre diseases. What I've found is that the peak experiences have to do with just performing well, being able to use my skills and experience, acting decisively and, God, correctly.

"The very best experience I've had here was getting through one particular afternoon. I had four patients in one hour. All of them had signs of cardiac failure. The resident was gone for some reason, or maybe we were between residents. Anyway, I remember clearly. I functioned perfectly. Two of the patients I had hospitalized immediately. I got them admitted without a doctor's signature, too. I just knew it was right and I couldn't get our doctor. The others I set up for tests, one with a cardiologist closer to his home, the other on a schedule of visits here. It was thorough, decisive. I felt great, just being able to do the right thing. Maybe it sounds dull, but it isn't. Oh, God, I was excited for days after that. Me. Indecisive old Janet.

"The people part..." Janet muses. "It varies so much. I don't feel impersonal, but you don't get involved emotionally. Not often. I remember a few weeks ago. It was funny. One afternoon I had this new patient. There was nothing special about him, a middle-aged man. But I just found myself liking him. I noticed myself interacting with him and I don't usually. We talked. He enjoyed me too. It was a real relationship and I remember being surprised that it was happening. He came in for a physical, minor aches and pains. Then I went up to find his X rays. They hadn't been sent down. I put the X ray up and flipped on the light switch. There was a tumor on his lung. My heart just stopped. He was a friend."

John is putting on his coat and Fred is waiting for him by the door. Janet starts to organize the clutter on her desk in preparation for leaving.

"So long, Janet," Fred says. "I've really enjoyed my rotation over here."

"Fred, same here," Janet smiles. "You're one of ... no, I can say really, you're the nicest resident we've had this year. Good luck in cardiology. John, you're coming for dinner on Christmas? Call me if you want a ride." The two men disappear down the hall.

"Someday," Janet says as she hangs up her lab coat, "I would like to live in the country. Get a couple of PAs and a doctor or two to form a rural clinic. Have a garden, things like that. It's not just a matter of sharing the work. It's getting away from the bad parts of this, the way the patients drift in and out. Most of them don't belong anywhere. They should belong somewhere."

SUMMARY

DUTIES: *Extends the services of a supervising physician by taking medical histories, doing physical examinations and, within circumscribed areas, diagnosing and treating patients. Most PAs are employed by primary care practices, although there are some programs that train assistants for certain medical specialties. PAs are likely to be hired by rural practices and hospital outpatient clinics.*

PHYSICIAN'S ASSISTANT

TRAINING: *There are three different avenues for training: medical school-based programs, additional training for registered nurses and Medex programs. Applicants to a medical school program must have a health-related background. The training takes two years. Nurse practitioners, who also serve as PAs, are registered nurses who receive from two months' to two years' supplemental education in pediatrics, family medicine and so forth. Programs such as these are available at nursing schools. Medex programs train people with substantial medical experience, such as medical corpsmen from the armed services. The training takes one year. Each individual in a Medex program has a medical preceptor or sponsor who works with the medical school in training the practitioner and hiring her/him after the training is completed. A similar program, Primex, has been developed for registered nurses. Physician's assistants and Medex graduates practice under the license of their supervising physician. About forty states have now altered their medical practice acts to allow for this delegation of authority. Most of these states also require that applicants pass an examination developed by the National Commission on Certification of Physician's Assistants before such delegation is approved. Nurse practitioners, on the other hand, are licensed as nurses. State nurse practice acts have been slow in changing to take account of these expanded roles. What tasks a physician's assistant or nurse practitioner does in practice is determined, to a large extent, by what the supervising physician will allow them to do. For more information, contact:*

> *The Association of Physician's Assistant Programs*
> *2150 Pennsylvania Avenue NW*
> *Washington, D.C.   20037*
>
> *or*
>
> *American Nurse's Association*
> *2420 Pershug Road*
> *Kansas City, Missouri   64108*

SALARY: *$12,000–25,000 depending on experience and location.*

2

HOME
HEALTH
AIDE

The Staff of the Hamilton County Visiting Nurse Association drifts into the new brick office building it shares with an insurance agency. Against one wall of the meeting room is a metal rack filled with brightly colored pamphlets: *What You Need to Know About VD, Care of Your Colostomy, The Facts of Emphysema, How to Qualify for Food Stamps, Techniques for the Baby Bath.*

Laurie Miller picks up a cup of coffee on her way into the staff room. She is twenty-four, a tall slender woman with curly red hair and freckles. She is wearing a light-blue cotton skirt with a matching tunic top, nylons, and sturdy shoes. "We are supposed to dress like this." She wrinkles her nose. "I don't see what's wrong with blue jeans, but some say it's an insult to the patients."

There are five registered nurses who work for the visiting nurse association. Laurie was the first home health aide to be hired. "We work essentially the way a nurse's aide does," she explains. "But we work more independently because we have to go out on our own. I came here because I needed a job. I went to an employment office. The visiting nurse association hires through them rather than having a lot of phone calls here. The only requirement was a high-school education and a car of your own. I had just graduated from college actually, in physical education. I couldn't teach though, because all the jobs needed other minors. No one needed a phys ed teacher. They all wanted a phys ed teacher who could also teach physics or home ec or something. This was the only job I could find.

"Since I was the first home health aide the agency hired, they really took a lot of care in training me. I spent a month or so just going around with them, studying the home health aide book, getting demonstrations on various procedures, before I did anything on my own. I don't think they were as thorough with the other two aides they've hired since." A large blond woman, Judy Arnold, greets Laurie.

"Are you seeing Mrs. Nemecek today?" she asks.

"Yes, I'm going there first."

"Well, her husband is gone for the day and her daughter won't be home until supper time. It would be good if one of us could go back this afternoon, to help her get to the bathroom and check up on her."

"OK. If I can't get to it, I'll ask Tony. He wanted to see her sometime soon anyway."

Several of the nurses and aides are at a big green blackboard, writing down their patient schedules for the day before they leave. Tony Mark, the agency's first male nurse, is finishing.

"Tony, would you have time to see Mrs. Nemecek this afternoon? You said you wanted to check the bandage sometime and she's going to be alone all day."

"I could stop by around three."

"That would be perfect. I'm on my way over there now." Laurie finishes writing down her list of patients for the day and picks up a small, black leather bag of supplies. "I probably won't even need this today, but I like to take it along in case." In her car, Laurie makes a note in a mileage log.

Mrs. Nemecek's house is in an older neighborhood of small houses with neat window boxes and clipped lawns. Laurie walks in the front door without knocking.

"Mrs. Nemecek, good morning."

"Oh, good morning, dear," a voice comes from a back room. The house is darkened by the large shade trees. It is full of furniture, but neat. Little tables display family pictures and souvenirs from family trips. Mrs. Nemecek is lying on a single bed in a corner of what was once a dining room. She has on a clean pink robe. She is about sixty, dark-haired, fastidiously groomed. Her hands, lying at her side, are bent and twisted with advanced arthritis.

"When I first started seeing Mrs. Nemecek, she had an ulcerated bedsore on her back that was unbelievable, wasn't it, Mrs. Nemecek?"

"Oh, it was awful. Well, I didn't get up for three years really.

Oh, they could lift me to go for rides and things like that but I was always in pain because of that sore."

"Anyway, we've been visiting her every day for five months. First we got the bedsore cleared up. Then we called in a physical therapist to do an evaluation. Her body had degenerated so badly because of the arthritis, she couldn't even sit up by herself. What else couldn't you do, Mrs. Nemecek?"

"I couldn't do anything, really. I couldn't comb my hair or pick anything up at all."

"So the physical therapist set up a regimen of exercises for her and now she can sit up, and before her daughter's wedding in August, she's going to be standing up by herself too. Right?"

"Well," Mrs. Nemecek laughs. "We're going to try."

"OK. Let's do those leg lifts first." Laurie takes a small weighted bag out of her kit and puts it on Mrs. Nemecek's right leg. "OK. Lift, 2-3-4-, 2-2-3-4-, 3-2-3-4-. Good. Getting a little shaky? Let's try the other one." The routine includes exercises for both legs, both arms and the chest.

"So your husband ran off to see the Chicago Cubs, huh?"

"Oh yes," Mrs. Nemecek laughs. "Oh, he was so happy he could go. It was so good for him to get away, and Janie could come and stay with me. He just loves the Cubs."

"Did you eat some breakfast? What'd you have?"

"The usual. Cereal and coffee and a hard-boiled egg."

"And she's left you some lunch here. Let's see what you're having. This doesn't look like very much." Laurie pokes into the foil wrapped paper plate by the bed.

"It's apricots and a sandwich and a candy bar. And I've got my water here."

"Are you sure that's enough? She won't be home until 5:30. Your diet says you can have two sandwiches."

"Oh, this is plenty."

"Well, at least you're not eating peanut butter again."

"Oh, I do love peanut butter. I know it's not good for me."

"OK. Let's check this dressing on the knee and then we'll get your brace on so you can go to the bathroom before I leave."

There is a small gauze bandage around the woman's knee where her brace had rubbed. The knee has a large white scar down the top from an operation for arthritis several years before. Laurie gets

HOME HEALTH AIDE

Mrs. Nemecek's brace on and helps her stand. With the brace and crutches Mrs. Nemecek makes her way to the bathroom. Then she takes a little walk around the house.

"Oh, that feels much better," she says. "Now I think I can get settled down." Laurie has the bed straightened and a fresh towel under the center. She helps the woman get down and undoes the brace for her.

"How are the skillets working?" Laurie points to two flat aluminum frying pans next to the bed.

"Oh, they're just fine. I just can't handle a regular bedpan, but these are so nice and flat and with the handle I really don't have much trouble."

"Whose idea was that?"

"Well, my husband. We kind of thought of it together."

"Don't let me forget your lunch now." Laurie places the paper plate back next to the bed. "I'm always afraid I'm going to go off and leave you without your lunch. I'll get you some fresh ice water now too. It's going to be kind of warm today."

Laurie comes back with a plastic pitcher tinkling with ice.

"Not too full dear. I spill. Yes, that's fine. Thank you."

"Now, are you all set? You got your telephone ready to go?"

"Oh yes. Glen offered to get me one of those little TV sets but I don't think there's much good on. I've got a lot of family in town so I just get on the phone and chat."

"OK. Tony is going to stop by this afternoon, but if you run into problems before then, you just call the office."

"Thank you, dear. Good-bye now." Laurie closes the door firmly as she leaves. Back in her car, she notes her mileage in the log book.

"There is a crucial difference between being an aide in a hospital and being an aide in a person's home. I mean, in a person's home, you have to go along with the style . . . you can't say 'This is right—this is the way things are done.' Last year I had this great old lady—she'd been a vegetarian for a long time and had all kinds of health magazines around. We just looked after her a bit, gave her a bath and made sure she was eating. Sometimes she ate unusual combinations, like avocados and bananas all mixed up. She kept her shoes in the oven too, to keep them warm, I think. We'd say 'Vida, you're going to start a fire.' We'd tell her family it was dangerous, but when it came down to it, she was still the boss. So her shoes stayed in the oven."

Fred Ames is Laurie's next patient. He is due for a weekly bath. In his eighties, Fred lives in a modern two-bedroom apartment in a student neighborhood. His sister, Alice, who's also in her eighties, lives with him. They moved off the farm two years ago. Fred greets Laurie from the couch, where he sits, smiling, in his farm overalls.

"Fred!" Laurie says. "Have you got long underwear on today? It's eighty-five degrees out!" Fred nods and smiles. He had surgery for cancer of the throat ten years earlier and has a hole in his throat through which he breathes. "Well, for heaven's sake. You are a stitch." Fred is already taking off his shoes in preparation for his bath. He had a mild stroke a year ago and is too unsteady to get in and out of the tub by himself.

"Fred has always lived with us, with my husband and myself," Alice says crisply. "We hadn't moved here yet. We had sold the farm but we hadn't actually moved yet when my husband died. I always wondered whether he would make it off the farm. He didn't." She is sitting in a sturdy old oak rocking chair with hand-sewn pillows on the back. It looks out of place in the imitation-wood paneled room. "Some people who were starting a radio station were real anxious to get our farm . . . That south forty acres was perfect, they said. Now sometimes I sit in here and listen to the radio and I think where that sound is coming from. Used to be the only sound from that field was the sound of corn hitting the wagons when Fred and I were picking. And my husband cursing the horses." She laughs.

After Fred's bath, Laurie leaves and goes back to the office to do some paper work.

"Fred was really embarrassed the first time I went to help him. But he's no problem now. A lot of older people worry about their bowels. Fred took laxatives all the time, even when he had diarrhea. As a result he sometimes had accidents. Once he did in the bathtub and I had to start all over. But we got the nurses to take the laxatives away, and Alice keeps them now. He only gets them once a day.

"I have a good case load now, everyone is nice . . . pretty cheerful. You get some grouchy ones sometimes, some fussy ones. Part of the job is trying not to let it get to you personally. I had a woman with a stroke once who did a lot of screaming. She was in her eighties and lived with her common-law husband and a son who drank a lot. He'd be drunk when I got there at nine o'clock. The woman should have been in a nursing home but the son tried to block it. Finally the court had her placed in a home. Those cases you just have to get in, do the best you can, and get out."

During the time between patients, Laurie and the other aides help with the paper work, sterilize equipment and do some typing and filing.

"The nurses have more paper work than we do," Laurie explains. "They have all the Medicaid and Medicare forms and county papers . . . it's endless. We charge for services on a sliding scale. The nurses have to get the income information, which can be kind of awkward. I'm glad we don't do that. It would make for a better relationship with the patients if they had a special person to do that. It bothers people to give that information out."

At noon time Laurie drives up to the main part of town to have a sandwich. Then she heads for a bookstore, to do an errand for one of her afternoon patients.

"Will you take this check?" she asks the cashier. "She's already signed it for the books. She said she'd called." The clerk nods and hands her two big books. Laurie takes the books and drives across town to an older duplex.

"The young woman in here has a slipped disc. She's supposed to be in bed except for going to the bathroom. She should be in bed for a month or two." Laurie knocks on the front door and calls softly.

"Jane? It's Laurie."

"OK." Jane is lying in bed, propped up with pillows. An Irish setter lifts his head lazily. Two cats are curled at the bottom of the bed. There is a stack of books on a bedside table.

"I brought the books. I'll get the dishes done for you. Is there anything else you'd like me to do?"

"The kitty litter, if you could," Jane says.

Laurie goes about her work quietly. Jane picks up the new books and looks through them. Laurie finishes her work quickly and heads for the door.

"So long Jane, see you tomorrow."

"Thanks," Jane says, but doesn't look up.

Back in the car, Laurie shrugs. "That's a difficult case. We're not supposed to do housekeeping. There are homemakers who are available from another office for that. But she has a medical problem and sometimes there is a fine line between the jobs, so I just do what I can to help out.

"We have a list of procedures that we're allowed to do as home health aides. The doctor has to approve having a home health aide in the home. The nurse approves the procedures. Our instructions include personal care such as baths, dressing, skin care. We also can assist with exercises and medications, food preparation and feeding. Light cleaning, like doing dishes and straightening up the patient's room, can be included. It depends on what the nurse assigns to us. If a procedure isn't on the list for a particular patient, we don't do it. We're not even allowed to cut toenails. You might be dealing with a diabetic patient where it could be really dangerous."

Laurie pulls the car over to the curb in front of a three-story brick office building in the main shopping area of town. An insurance agency and a gift shop are downstairs. Sarah Harris lives on the second floor.

"Well, I'm five minutes early. That means I watch the end of "The Secret Storm." That's her favorite TV show. She won't talk to me until it's over."

Laurie opens the kitchen door of the second-floor apartment and walks through a dark old-fashioned kitchen. Sarah is sitting in a big living room with windows on three sides.

The afternoon light filters through the lace curtains that hang from ceiling to floor. A fake fireplace is at one end of the room. A china closet with glass doors houses a collection of fine crystal goblets, and a ceramic Hawaiian girl in a grass skirt. Sarah is about sixty-five.

"Almost over?" Laurie asks.

"Watch this, honey. There's a wedding." Organ music comes from the direction of the television. "Sandy and Michael are finally getting married. Even though he has the trial ahead. Oh, don't weddings make you want to cry?"

"How are you feeling today, Sarah? You look pretty tired."

"Oh, I spent the morning cleaning the refrigerator. See, those are his daughters. Aren't they cute?"

"Why didn't you wait for someone to help you? You can't be doing that heavy work now. I'll bet you're too tired to go for a walk."

"Oh, I'm not walking today. I really am tired."

Laurie seats herself in a stuffed chair next to Sarah.

"Well, I shouldn't have bothered to come. Did you get your lunch?"

"Oh yes. It was pretty good too, today. I didn't care for the jello. See the maid-of-honor there? She's thinking about getting back with her husband. Shoot."

"Shall I turn it off now?"

"Yeah. Go ahead. It's over. Say, are you coming tomorrow?"

"Well, one of the nurses may be coming instead tomorrow, to check up on my care. You still want to get your sister something?"

"Yup."

"Well, I'll come take you the next day. Are you using your cane?"

"I'm getting around on it all right now."

"Listen, as long as you're too tired to get out, I'm going to run along. I'll be back day after tomorrow and we'll go out."

"OK. Sorry I'm not good company today, but I'm bushed."

"See you later."

On the way out, Laurie passes an open door to another apartment. Inside, an old man rocks methodically in a stuffed rocker. A grey-haired woman lies asleep on a day bed next to a fan.

"That's a brother and sister. They're both seen by the nurses." Laurie explains, "He's blind. The Meals on Wheels comes to them too . . . I don't think they go out at all."

"Sarah Harris has multiple sclerosis," Laurie explains as she drives back toward the office. "She found out just before she was going to retire. She was a secretary for years. It was hard on her at first, but she's adjusted really well. She's so chipper sometimes it really makes you feel humble."

At the edge of town, Laurie stops in front of a little white house, badly in need of paint.

"Sam is ninety-four," Laurie says as she walks up the steps. "He burned his back because he didn't rinse a bleached shirt out properly. I put cream on his back every day for the burns. Other than that, he's on his own pretty much."

"Well, hi." It is Sam's daughter, a nervous, heavyset woman who greets Laurie at the door. "Honestly, I've been so worried. He won't answer the phone. I try to get over every day, but it would be nice if he'd answer the damn phone, you know?"

"I can't hear it with the TV," Sam says. He is toothless, his voice a bit muffled. He has short silver hair, and wears a sleeveless T-shirt.

"Well, put it over next to you," Laurie scolds. "You've got to be where people can reach you, Sam." She takes a surgical glove from her bag and puts it on. "Get your shirt up. Now, that's it." The cream she uses is laid out on a bookcase by Sam's chair.

"Here," Sam offers a bottle to Laurie from out of a paper bag next to his chair. "Have some."

"No, Sam, you know I can't drink that. Apricot brandy? Who brought you that? Bill?"

"Yup."

"Well, that's real nice."

"I used to drive for a lady doctor," Sam says, looking out the window. "Horse and wagon. Down in Kirksville, Missouri. She was the bravest person I ever saw. One night we were headed back and we seen a cyclone coming up in the back. 'Come on, Sam,' she said. 'Let's race this thing.' So we did. We went right past houses that had been tore up and everything. We made it home. Those horses were so lathered up you could scrape it right off."

"I'm not feeling so well myself," Sam's daughter says. "I wish I didn't have to worry about him so, Laurie."

"Well, listen. You have the office phone. You call the office when you can't reach him. One of us is always scooting around. We can pop in on him, if he's too stubborn to move the phone two feet. I'll see you tomorrow, Sam."

Laurie goes back to the office before her last visit for the day and finishes filling out the day's papers. Once finished she heads south, where the city drops suddenly into corn and soybean fields. She turns off the highway onto a county road. The farms are immaculately groomed.

Laurie greets Mrs. Frank, an elderly woman in a small modern house. The woman has a blood clot in her leg and badly swollen legs. Laurie gives her a sponge bath, helps her into a clean gown, puts her in a wheelchair and moves her into the living room. Laurie brushes her long grey hair and does it into a braid for her. She does this, chatting with the woman and with the two granddaughters who are visiting.

It is late afternoon when Laurie leaves Mrs. Frank. Mr. Frank is watering the flowers in front of the house as she passes.

"Never water in the noon sun," he says.

"Right!" Laurie calls back as she gets in her car.

Laurie heads toward the house she shares with another woman. "That lady has plenty of family to take care of her. But it's good to have some outside help. It helps keep the sick person from becoming quite such a chore . . . I mean the family knows I'm going to be there to do certain things. They can relax a bit.

"I had never been around a sick person before I took this job. No one was ever sick in my house. I'd never been in the hospital. Just sprains from sports. This job really depressed me at first. Sick people can be a drag. Everyone has these big problems. You just feel overwhelmed. Then gradually, you learn to do your thing, to treat them like people, and not like problems. I don't want to stay in this job forever. But I can see the possibilities. No, I never would have considered a health career before, but I can see it as a real possibility now."

SUMMARY

DUTIES: *Provides home management, grooming and simple patient care services to patients in their own homes, under the supervision of a registered nurse and a physician. This includes assisting the patient in bathing, grooming, exercise, evaluating the patient's condition and nutritional status, making the patient's bed and doing light housekeeping.*

TRAINING: *High-school graduate or equivalent. Some junior colleges provide training programs and most employers provide training for applicants.*

SALARY: *$6,000–10,000 depending on location.*

3.

EMERGENCY MEDICAL TECHNICIAN

John Spencer arrives for the night shift a little before eleven. Mike and George, the evening shift emergency medical technicians (EMT), are watching the last inning of the baseball game with some of the firemen in the station house. They sip cokes with their feet up on the table, trading commentaries on the game. Most of the firemen in the city are older than the EMTs. The average age of the EMTs in the city is about twenty-four. There has been some friction between the two groups in some of the other firehouses, even a couple of fist fights between individuals with short tempers. The firemen are a little jealous of the new group and sometimes the EMTs are just a little too young and cocky. But, at Firehouse 6, everybody is on friendly terms.

"Hi, what's been happening?" John asks.

"Oh, nothing very exciting. Took a couple of runs to the hospital. Just people who needed to see a doctor who didn't have transportation. There was an accident on the expressway during rush hour, a fender bender. A couple of people with bad bruises that had to be taken to be X-rayed. Nothing serious. Must be about time for a big one and looks like you're the lucky man," Mike says, smiling.

"Thanks a lot," John laughs.

"Being an emergency medical technician isn't like the television show," John explains. "Most of the time you're just cooling your heels waiting. We get about ten or twelve calls a day to this station, most of them routine. We're lucky to get two or three big ones in a month, ones where we really get a chance to use our skills in saving a life. Every time a call comes in, you find yourself hoping it's one of those big ones. The firemen think we've got all the glamour and prestige. Well, we'll just try to encourage that thinking."

"Aw, but remember last month," Mike counters, "when those trucks jacknifed on the expressway and rolled down the embankment and we had to pull the people out with extension ladders and ropes? That sure as hell would have made a great 'Emergency' episode."

"Come on, Mike, no war stories tonight. Save them for your book," John yawns. "Whenever EMTs get together they retell the war stories about the big ones where they really had to perform. Mike is going to write a book about it. Ever since that guy in New York wrote the best seller about his fire company, Mike's been busy taking notes."

"OK fella, let's see who's laughing when you see me on the Johnny Carson Show," Mike says.

They all laugh.

John's background is a little different from the others. Some are attracted by the lights and sirens. They're young and they want adventure. John was a biology major in college.

"I was interested in medicine, so I figured getting into emergency medical care wouldn't hurt. I helped organize a volunteer ambulance service in the suburb where I lived. I didn't have the grades for medical school, so, when the city's program started up, I applied. Now it's getting harder to get in. A lot of junior colleges are starting up two-year programs for paramedics.

"Now I spend a lot of time helping to train the new recruits. They need a basic knowledge of emergency medicine and patient-care skills. Besides that, there are two things they have to be able to do to make it. First, they have to know how to read street maps. In real emergencies a minute or so makes all the difference. If you make a couple of wrong turns or end up fumbling around trying to find a street address on a map, it doesn't make any difference how much you know about emergency medical treatment, it won't do any good. Second, you've got to be able to relate to the people and understand what they're going through. You've got to be in control of the situation. You can't afford to get flustered and rush around trying to find the things that you need."

John has completed all of the specialized training to be an EMT. Several years ago, he completed the EMT I program. It includes

80 hours of classroom instruction that covers basic first aid, CPR (cardiopulmonary resuscitation), treatment of various medical emergencies and extrication of individuals trapped in automobile accidents. He has also just completed the EMT II or paramedic program that includes over 200 hours of classroom and clinical instruction. They were taught how to start IVs and the types of emergency drugs to use with them, how to defibrillate a heart attack victim through electroshock, how to read electrocardiograms and identify the key patterns, how to treat shock. They even learned how to assist in the delivery of a baby.

John took the state certification exam that contained 150 multiple choice questions several months ago and passed.

"Prehospital emergency care is a very specialized area. I doubt many physicians could pass the certification exam except, of course, those who have specialized in emergency medicine or new medical school grads. It is not that complicated, though. There are only about twenty drugs that are used in emergency situations and you need to know how to administer them, and what the indications and countraindications are for each. Most of the drugs are used in treating a cardiac victim. There are a limited number of things you can do immediately that make any difference in saving a person's life, but the technology is constantly changing. We can keep up with it, because our concerns are so specialized. For example, we're using drugs in the field that were experimental five years ago. Space-age technology led to the development of portable heart monitors and defibrillators. Ten years ago it was just impractical because of the weight and size of the equipment.

"We used to have a problem preventing vomit from blocking the airways of a victim. There's a procedure for doing this in a hospital called tracheal intubation, but it requires some skill and physicians didn't want to delegate that task to paramedics in the field. A new device was recently developed as an alternative, called an esophageal opturator. The paramedic can blindly insert the tube with an inflatable cuff down the pharynx and into the esophagus. When inflated, it blocks the esophagus, preventing aspiration from the stomach (vomit) from entering the lungs while still permitting air to be passed into them.

"It's easy to fool yourself and think you know more than you do. A lot of people in the emergency rooms get irritated with some EMTs. I mean, the nurses have four years of training and still haven't been trained to give IVs and here we are, after six months, giving intravenous medications and all. Most of the stuff we learn is taught to nurses in a specialized intensive-care program after they have received an RN degree.

"Yet, you know, if I had a heart attack, there's no question that I'd rather have an EMT than a doctor. EMTs see more fresh heart attacks in a year than most physicians see in their whole lives. I can remember one situation where I actually ended up directing the emergency room staff. As we were dropping a patient off in the emergency room, a patient in cardiac arrest arrived by volunteer ambulance. The nurse tried to start an IV in the patient's wrist even though there were all kinds of possibilities in the antecubical space (inside surface of the elbow joint). The physician was just standing there, waiting. Finally, I asked if they would mind if I tried and I got the IV started immediately. I told the physician that it might be a good idea to start giving the patient two ampules of sodium bicarbonate since the patient had been in arrest for more than thirty minutes. He said, 'It might be a good idea to go ahead,' but he was more interested in looking at the EKG which, of course, picked up all the interference from doing CPR. The patient was dead by that time."

Jack, John's partner on the night shift, arrives. The two have been working together for about a year. They work well together. Jack is a Vietnam veteran medical corpsman. Nothing seems to faze him. He moves at the same even pace no matter what is happening, keeping up a quiet banter, but everything that needs to be accomplished gets done very quickly.

The two evening shift EMTs leave and Jack and John are left in the now quiet firehouse sipping coffee.

"You know, it all can be pretty dull at times," Jack says. "But every time the dispatcher rings, it does something for me. You never know quite what it's going to be. I perform best under that kind of pressure. I thrive on it."

Half an hour later the dispatcher's phone rings. Jack gets the message as John starts the van. They pull out with the lights flashing. John touches the siren as they ease through a red light.

"716 North 23rd Street. Bet somebody's OD'd again," Jack says.

"No contest," John sighs. "After a while, you get to know the city pretty well. You see parts of it that most people never see. Not just the families with the two kids and the three-bedroom ranch house. You see places that haven't been cleaned in years, with rotting food and the smell of urine and crap in the bedrooms. You see old guys covering themselves up with newspapers to keep warm in a back alley filled with garbage, nursing a lousy bottle of wine."

The apartment is on the third landing. The hallway has a dark musty odor. The door to the apartment is ajar. There is a young, thin, dark-haired woman lying under the table motionless. Everyone else has disappeared, apparently in a hurry. There are still several cigarettes burning in the ashtray on the table. Jack quickly performs an examination. Her breathing is shallow and slow. Her pupils are constricted. There's no alcohol on her breath and she doesn't react to pricks on her hand with a pin. Jack looks closely at the purple needle marks on her arm.

"Medic Command. This is Medic 3."

"Go ahead, Medic 3, this is Command." The voice is that of a physician in a nearby hospital emergency room.

"We have a twenty-five-year-old female patient, unconscious, unresponsive to verbal and painful stimuli. There are signs of recent needle marks and drug paraphernalia present at the scene. Her vital signs are the following: pulse 98, blood pressure 110/80, pupils constricted and non-reactive, respiration of 12 and very shallow. We're administering O_2 via mask at eight liters per minute and transporting her to Suburban General with an ETA (estimated time of arrival) of fifteen minutes."

"This is Medic Command, Dr. Smith. Start an IV D5W (5 percent Dextrose and water) KVO (Keep Valve Open) and administer .4 milligrams of Narcan IV, push, slowly, monitoring respiration. Get back to me if any complications arise." John starts the IV and Jack begins to slowly inject the Narcan.

"Narcan is a narcotic antagonist. It works well and there are no side effects so it's pretty safe to use. The only thing you have to worry about is that it works too fast and you pull somebody out of their sixty-dollar high. Sometimes they're mad as hell at you for ruining their trip and want to beat you up."

A few minutes later, the woman moans and stirs.

"OK, you've had a bad one. We're going to take you to the hospital to be checked out."

The woman nods, her eyes are wide open, frightened. She doesn't speak.

They put her on the litter, wrap her in a blanket and carry her to the van.

As they bring her into the emergency entrance of the hospital, they get a second call over their radio. Someone who lives on the other side of the expressway needs assistance. Quickly, they move the woman out of the van and onto a stretcher. They leave her by the admission desk and head across town for their next emergency.

When they arrive at the small home, a man is lying on the living room couch, wincing with pain and clutching his stomach. His wife hovers in the background.

"It's all right, Martha. You're such a worry wart. It's just the ulcers acting up again. Just give me some warm milk." John examines the man but finds that his examination isn't conclusive. The medical command requests his transfer to the hospital for observation.

"No way. I'm going to stay right here," the man says. "You're not going to stick me in the hospital. We've got enough money troubles."

The wife pleads with him, but he refuses.

After making their own effort to reason with him, Jack and John finally shrug their shoulders and leave.

"It's a tough situation," John explains. "We can't take a person to the hospital without her or his consent. He's probably right about the ulcer, but you always worry about these things. I remember one call we got last year. The wife called. The man was having congestive heart failure, but refused to go with us. His wife pleaded with us to take him, but we couldn't. We got a call back the next day to the same address, a probable DOA (dead on arrival). When the dispatcher says that to you, you can be pretty sure they're dead. When we got there, the husband was sitting at the kitchen table, his eyes open, slumped a bit. He'd been like that for twelve hours. He was dead."

They drive back slowly to the station. The streets are empty. They listen to the police band on their radio. Things are quiet.

In the station house, they both sit sipping instant coffee. Jack decides to take a catnap on a cot in the lounge. Out of habit, John systematically checks over the supplies in the van.

"We change shifts every month. Last month, I was on the evening shift. It's a little hard to get used to. You find yourself going out for pizza and beer after work at 8:00 a.m."

The ambulances are modified vans. The roofs are raised two feet and they are lengthened an additional two feet to meet federal guidelines. Emergency vehicles must have a tile floor. The main stretcher lies along the driver's side of the van. Above it are clear plastic cabinets that contain most of the smaller equipment that is needed—drugs, bandages, syringes. On the other side are long benches where the EMT sits to work on the patient. Underneath the bench the heavy equipment is stored—the splints, extra blankets, ropes, the hydraulic jacks and metal cutting equipment used in extricating victims of automobile accidents. At the front end of the compartment there is a jump seat just behind where the patient's head rests. A large cylinder of oxygen is strapped to the wall. The suction equipment, which operates off of the van's engine, and the oxygen can be used on the patient from the jump seat. There is a small passageway to the front of the van. Both the back and the front of the van are equipped with radios.

Another call comes in from the dispatcher. John and Jack are directed to a high-rise apartment five minutes away. At the scene, the mother is weeping, pulling at her hair. A nine-year-old boy is lying on his bed with his mouth open, having great difficulty breathing. His face is slate blue and his eyes are wide open.

"This is Medic 3 to Command. We have a nine-year-old boy, cyanotic, experiencing extreme difficulty in breathing. He is a chronic asthmatic and is taking the following medication . . ." John rattles off the rest of the history.

"OK, Medic 3, this is Command, Doctor Spencer. Administer low concentration of O_2 via nasal cannula (tube) and .2 milligrams Epinephrine I.M. (intramuscular)."

Within five minutes the boy is breathing more easily, normal color has returned to his face and he wants to walk to the ambulance rather than be carried on the stretcher.

"Everything's going to be fine, Billy," his mother says. The mother rides in the van with the boy; the father and the older son follow behind in their car.

"Hi, John," the nurse says. "Bring him right into this cubicle. Dr. Morris will be right down." The doctor arrives, glares at them silently, and the two EMTs leave. Heading back toward the fire station, John talks about how the doctors feel about EMTs.

"Our relationship with some of the medical staff of that hospital is a little cool. They've had bad experiences with some of the volunteer ambulance drivers. You know, they've got a lot of siren-crazy kids who think that, because they've had a first-aid course, they can start ordering people around. They make some bad mistakes occasionally. There's just no way that they can get the kind of experience that we get. But the hospital people who can distinguish between us and the volunteers have a lot of respect for what we do. Treating patients in the field is a lot different from doing it in a brightly lit, well-equipped hospital. They appreciate the difficulties we face.

"But, you know, it works both ways. I've seen a lot of times when the medical staffs in hospitals have made bad mistakes too. I remember once, about a year ago, we had a female patient we found in cardiac arrest in her bedroom at four in the morning. After starting an IV, defibrillating and administering some drugs, she started to respond. She was responding much better on the way to the hospital but, just as we got to the entrance she aspirated and went into cardiac arrest. I rushed her into the emergency room and the two residents on duty took one look at her, shrugged their shoulders and pulled a sheet over her face.

" 'You can't do that,' I yelled at them. 'Not after I've spent an hour reviving her.' I really lost my cool. One of the doctors stayed watching from the doorway while the other two left. I started working on her frantically. I suctioned her out and got the physician to intubate her. We got her heart started again and in twenty minutes she'd got some color back and wasn't looking so much like a corpse. Three weeks later they discharged her. I get letters from her every now and then.

"You really can't blame the interns though. If you bring someone in cyanotic, without pulse or respiration, after going out forty-five minutes earlier to pick them up, it's pretty easy to jump to the conclusion that they're stone cold dead. You only have four or five minutes to get the heart started again before there's permanent brain damage. Sometimes it works the other way too, you know, practice time for the interns and residents. They work over somebody so everybody gets a chance to practice even though they know there's no chance that the person will pull through."

They back up quietly to their firehouse portal.

"It's a kind of delicate relationship we have with the physicians in the emergency room. We use them for our 'medical command.' Some EMTs can only defibrillate a heart attack victim once without medical orders. Everything else we do has to come from the physician orders. It's really a polite fiction that's maintained. Each emergency room of a hospital which gives orders to paramedics has a manual that tells what we're supposed to do, given what we report from the scene. We provide the information about the patient to the physician, she or he interprets the information and has us initiate a form of care. We know what the physician is going to say for a given situation and we can control what she or he tells us by the way we present the patient's symptoms.

"On that television show, 'Emergency,' they make a big thing about radio transmittal of EKGs to the physician. Most people recognize that we can do as good a job in interpreting the EKGs. We're only concerned with life-threatening arrhythmias that need immediate attention in terms of anti-arrhythmia drugs or counter shock. Also, most of the monitors have only three leads. A physician needs twelve leads to do diagnostic work. We have the capability of transmitting EKGs by telephone but it's rarely used. Most physicians have learned to trust our judgment."

They drink some more instant coffee and a half-hour passes before the next call comes from the dispatcher. He instructs them to drive to the other side of town. When they arrive at the small, shabby row house, an elderly woman greets them. Her sister has had a high fever for several days. She wants to get her to an emergency room to have a doctor look at her. She's afraid.

"You know this is not really an emergency and you could get a private ambulance to move her," John explains. "We don't want to tie up the emergency vehicles this way."

The woman is insistent and so John shrugs and moves. He helps put the woman on the litter.

"Don't worry, everything's going to be fine," John tells the woman.

They drive across town to the public hospital and talk quietly in the front compartment about the situation.

"There's really no need for us to do this. It's not an emergency situation, but they probably don't have the money to pay for a private ambulance. We could refuse but suppose she really gets sick later. We'd be in a terrible mess, so it's better just to be on the safe side. It's the most frequent kind of call we get. People who just need transportation to a hospital or a doctor."

"Oh, well, anything's better than the suicides," Jack says. "I have a hard time taking them. You never know whether you're going to find a corpse or a man waiting to shoot you. Everyone's different. I remember finding one guy who had hung himself in a mobile trailer park. His trailer ceiling was too low, so he drove a nail into the ceiling, attached his belt to it and lifted up his legs so they wouldn't touch the floor. He was dead."

"I don't know," John says. "Sometimes the auto accidents can really get to me. There's a stretch of the freeway here that has killed ten people in the last year. Somehow, after they go under the overpass they lose control. I remember one kid who had been drinking crashed into the side of the overpass. We had a devil of a time getting him free. Couldn't figure out what was holding him in. He was slumped up under the dashboard. We couldn't pull him free. Then I realized that his right thigh was impaled on the metal part of the brake pedal. We had to cut the pedal with a saw and transport him to the hospital with it in place."

Arriving at the hospital, they leave the woman and her sister at the admission desk. As they head back to the station house, grey-yellow light is beginning to brighten the eastern sky. Just as the red sun edges over the horizon they get a call from the dispatcher.

"60th and Main, man unconscious."

The lights flash as they pick up speed on the empty streets.

There is a motionless figure sprawled against the curb. Several people are standing next to him poking at him gingerly. They step back as the van pulls up. John feels his pulse and checks his respiration. He's alive. The figure begins to stir.

"What's the problem?" John asks.

"Nothing, nothing, it's OK, I'll go." The man's speech is slurred. A bottle stuffed in a bag falls from a tattered pocket and clatters to the pavement. He has a week's growth of whiskers on his face, a few rotten, yellow teeth and a large dark bruise on his head. He tries to stand up but he can't.

"OK, take it easy, don't move. We've got a stretcher for you." They are told by medical command to bring him into the hospital for observation.

They lift him gently onto the stretcher, cover him with a blanket and put him inside the van.

"You have to be very careful with drunks," John says. "It could be an uncontrolled diabetic or a stroke victim. Sometimes they get hit by cars. I remember picking up one guy once who claimed he was fine and wanted to walk home when he actually had a fractured pelvis and ruptured spleen."

It is seven in the morning by the time they get back to the firehouse. John showers and changes into his street clothes. Jack motions to him with his hand as if he were drinking a can of beer.

"Not this time, Jack. I'm just going to go home and sack out," John says. He waves to the two day-shift EMTs in the lounge and heads for his car.

SUMMARY

DUTIES: *Provides emergency medical services in the field and transports patients to emergency rooms.*

TRAINING: *Metropolitan police and fire departments in most large cities have assumed responsibility for training EMTs. Individuals who have been working either as policemen or firemen can usually apply for this training after a year of employment. Some commercial ambulance companies also offer EMT training. Within police and fire departments there tends to be a high turnover of EMTs. They rise quickly in the ranks of their department, thus leaving their EMT assignments behind. A few junior colleges offer training programs in cooperation with city departments. A national examination must be passed for certification. For more information, contact local public agencies such as the police department, or:*

> *National Registry of EMTs*
> *P. O. Box 29233*
> *Columbus, Ohio   43229*

SALARY: *$7,500–9,000 to start.*

RELATED OCCUPATIONS

Since the related occupations for this section are not new or are not really independent occupations, they best fit into either of the two following sections: "New Jobs for Old Practitioners" or "Therapists and Technicians." Look over the chapters in these two sections and at the related occupations listed at the end of each section. These should give you some ideas about other possibilities for "new practitioners."

new jobs for old practitioners

. . . . .

The old practitioners used to include only a few occupations. The nurse, the doctor, the dentist and the local pharmacist made up the list of health workers that most people could name. In medicine today, there is no such thing as an old practitioner—a person who is doing the same job s/he did fifty years ago. The explosion of new health occupations has brought on a redefinition of the old ones. The osteopath presented in chapter 4 is a member of an old profession but his job has changed radically with new technology. Likewise, the midwife, a very old practitioner, has had her job reshaped by modern medical and counseling techniques.

Old practitioners are also entering the health care sector from other disciplines. Many new health-related jobs are opening up for people not traditionally associated with medicine. Physicists and engineers are developing specialties to assist with the technical challenges of medicine. Social workers have a medical branch which helps patients cope with their illnesses and with the health care system.

Another trend among the old practitioners has been toward increased specialization. Specialization has lured many doctors away from general practice and into the more prestigious and higher paying specialty areas. This has made primary care difficult to find and has meant that less populated areas, which cannot support specialists, have had trouble finding physicians to look after routine health problems. Some medical schools have addressed this problem by creating the Family Practice Physician (described at the end of this section). This has helped to fill, somewhat, the gap that specialization has created.

As with the health profession as a whole, the need for the old practitioners is expected to continue growing. This growth, however, will have to include both new specialists, such as the clinical pharmacist seen in this section, and new versions of primary care providers.

4

DOCTOR OF OSTEOPATHY

A two-lane highway leads into the midwestern town of Randall. On this July morning, the sun shimmers off broad leaves of corn, and bakes the newly cultivated ground between low rows of soybeans. Men still walk their bean fields here. They bring children, grandchildren or hired teenagers, and walk the rows, pulling up the weeds and volunteer corn that herbicides and cultivation have missed. It is a matter of pride to keep the bean fields clean of shaggy intruders. The farmer who plants his ground with $50,000 worth of machinery and a full line of agricultural chemicals, may still walk a forty-acre bean field with a hoe.

Dr. Herbert Grass practices in the town that starts ten feet from where the corn fields stop at the Randall grain elevator. Two thousand people live here, mostly in small white houses with neat gardens and porch swings. There are two modern developments at the edge of town. Dr. Grass has his office on Main Street. The sign says, "Dr. Herbert Grass, D.O." Doctor of Osteopathy.

"The osteopath has always got to prove himself," Dr. Grass explains. "The MD, whether he's good or bad, can present himself and have the world at his feet. The osteopath has got to prove himself. We have to take the same state board exams in order to practice, but the osteopath is still seen by a lot of people as a quack. That's a myth that's encouraged by the medics, by the MDs, that is."

Dr. Grass has practiced in Randall for almost ten years. "This town needed a doctor. I've built up my practice slowly, but I'm part of the town now. I meet all the medical needs here. The nursing homes, the football team in the fall, everything. Oh, I refer patients to doctors in the city, and I send them to the big hospitals when they need it. But I do an awful lot of medicine here. Before they send a doctor into a specialty area, they should make them work as a country GP. They'd learn to use their heads a little. You don't have fifty specialists to lean on here. You are it."

Dr. Grass is in his early fifties. He is heavyset, with dark hair and glasses. He wears a mint green doctor's tunic, plaid pants and white shoes. The office is newly paneled, with gold framed mirrors on the walls. There are six examining rooms, a large clerical area, an office for Dr. Grass, a lab and drug room and an X-ray room. "The closest X-ray machine is thirty miles away at a little hospital. It doesn't make sense, so I got one here. My assistants know how to use it." Dr. Grass has three women working for him. One of them handles the bookkeeping. The other two take blood pressures and histories from patients before he sees them, and do the standard lab tests and shots.

Ann stands next to him as she hands him a patient chart. "Melissa is here. She's talked to me about her mother and about putting her in the nursing home. You know she could move in with her mother, into one of the little apartments. But it seems if she does that, she won't qualify for the Title 19 money anymore because she'll have too much with only half the rent."

"Now here's a case," the doctor says. "We're just up to it in government red tape, trying to get some of the people served. Here's a woman who's sick, her mother is in her eighties. If you put them both together where they'd be happy, they'd lose all their money, even though it would be saving the government money. Then we have Charlie over there at the grain elevator. Had heart surgery. Two kids. $78 a month in drug expenses. We can't get aid to him for anything."

"And it just breaks your heart," Ann says. She is a well-groomed middle-aged woman. "You know there are people getting funds who don't need it nearly so bad."

Dr. Grass picks up Melissa's chart and walks into an examining room across the hall. Melissa is in her late fifties, a heavy woman with thin grey hair.

"Well, you're keeping your blood pressure down, Melissa," the doctor smiles. "No complaints?"

"No. I'm doing all right. This heat is gettin' to me, but I'm OK."

"How are you set for medication?" he asks as he reaches for a stethoscope hanging on the wall.

"Oh, I have a few more days."

"Deep breath. OK. Well, we'll get you set for another two weeks. Then we'll want to see you again. You seem to be fine. We'll take another look at that nursing home thing for your mother, too. This is getting ridiculous."

"Oh, I know that," Melissa smiles.

Ann is doing a urine test on another patient in the lab room.

"Ann, would you get Melissa another two weeks of her pills? In a small town like this," Dr. Grass explains, "you have to keep medications on hand. We have one drugstore, but it closes at five. If someone needs something in the night, they'd have to go thirty miles to get it if I didn't keep things here."

He picks up another chart in his office and goes to an examining room. A big blond man is sitting at the examining table. He has his six-year-old son with him. The man is wearing a navy blue work uniform with his name, "Ron," in red letters on the pocket. His heaviness makes him look older than his thirty-three years.

"Ron, the blood pressure is doing all right." Dr. Grass glances at the record the assistants have done. "But you're not doing much with the weight problem. Those pills cut your appetite at all?"

"Not much, I guess." Ron laughs, and reaches out to his boy's head.

"You working overtime on the gas truck?"

"Oh yeah. They've given me a whole new route down south of town now for the summer."

"Well, less time for beer drinking then. We'll try these pills another two weeks then, and keep up with the blood pressure medication."

"Say, Doc, is it natural for a kid to have a soft spot here?" Ron pushes the child's head gently toward the doctor. Dr. Grass feels the top of his head carefully.

"Oh yeah. That's OK. That's not a real soft spot."

"Well, that's what I told him. But he got in a fight with his brother and got dumped on his head. He thought that's when it happened."

"No, it'll stick together, Danny," Dr. Grass smiles and goes back to his office.

He takes a phone call while he lights a cigarette. "No, Fred. I think you did the right thing. That's it. OK." He hangs up. "I have another office in the next town, thirty miles away." He explains, "I have a physician's assistant, Fred, who got started there this week. They have a little hospital, so I see patients there in the afternoon. Then I come back here usually. It was getting too much. Quiet day like this I'll probably see fifty patients altogether. Have busy days where I see ninety or so."

An elderly gentleman is in an examination room. He has bib overalls on his tall slender frame. He shakes mildly, but steadily, from Parkinson's disease.

"Feeling kind of light headed, are you, Ralph?" Dr. Grass glances at a chart.

"Well, yes, I have last few days. Yesterday I was picking beans with the missus and when I stood up, I just felt real funny. Then a few times after that."

"How long does it last?"

"Oh, just a few minutes," Ralph says, as the doctor listens to his heart.

"Well, everything checks out all right. Blood pressure is good. No one can stand out in this ninety-degree heat and not feel a little dizzy. You should stay in during the heat of the day, Ralph. Never mind what Lucy says. Are you OK except for that?"

"Well, bowels been a little stubborn."

"You take a laxative?"

"Yes, I take it once a day."

"Well, that should do the trick. If this dizziness lasts much longer or gets any worse, you call me."

In the next room, a high school boy with a sprained ankle is waiting for a checkup. He is wearing a T-shirt with bar bells across the top and the words "Randall 1300 lb. Club."

"Still painful?" Dr. Grass says, turning the ankle gently. "The swelling is certainly down."

"Still hurts some," the boy says.

"Ann," Dr. Grass calls through the open door. "Would you put Randy on the magna therm? I use that machine a lot during football season. It's ultrasound and infrared heat treatment. That's the EKG machine there." He points to an examining room. "My assistants run the tests. We have a telephone hookup to a cardiologist in the city. I think I can give my patients pretty good care from this office. I think I practice good medicine here.

"Now, a few years back, the government said they wanted you to practice good medicine . . . Good diagnostic work is needed in good medicine. That's what they meant. Now they're going backwards, complaining about all the tests being done. They make liars out of the doctors. The insurance companies do too. You see, they don't want to pay for diagnostic tests. So you end up putting patients in the hospital to cover tests you know they can't afford. The government is just after you and after you. They're going to end up with socialized medicine and then they're going to find out how expensive medicine is. You think they're going to get some government doctor to work as hard as I do? No way.

"Oh, I've calmed down a lot," Dr. Grass goes on. "I used to be much more of a maverick than I am now. I was accepted into Indiana Medical School, you see. This was after World War II. I'd been an operating-room technician during the war. My father took sick in Joplin, Missouri. There were no MDs, just an osteopath. Well, he got such good care, he said, 'Herbert, why don't you look into this.' So I did. I got all the information. Classroom hours were longer for the DO. Surgical time was longer. It was really a more extensive education. This isn't true now; they've cut it down. But then it was longer. Then there is the added benefit of the osteopathic treatment, bone manipulation, that you learn. It's in the MD textbooks, but they don't actually teach it in the schools. I was dating a girl at the time whose father was an MD. He said, 'You'll have an extra technique to use on your patients as a DO, but you'll have to fight all your life to be accepted.'

"Well, I went ahead. And he was right. I don't know the exact history of the reputation. The man who started the first school for DOs in Kirksville, Missouri, was an MD. He could have given either an MD or a DO degree, but he was a renegade and wanted to separate himself from the MDs. They used to call osteopaths 'ten finger men' because of the manipulative therapy. That was before World War II. In World War II, in many areas of the country, all the MDs were taken, and DOs were all that were left. So people got to know the DO, got to know what he could do. Now there are places, in Michigan for example, where the DO has even more status than the MD. But there are a lot of quack accusations. The MDs don't mind that, by the way.

"Well, hell yes, you get paranoid. Now, two years ago I went to open up an office in the next town. They had a brilliant MD there, who was an alcoholic and going fast. Then they had a young couple, husband and wife MD team, moving in. Well, they say you should start by going to the bank when you open a practice in a new town. Take out a loan, even if you don't need it. So I went there with the lawyer who was going to rent me office space. 'Fine, fine,' the banker said. 'Yes, we need a doctor, you can have all the money you want.'

"So we talked and toward the end I said, 'You know I am a DO.' That banker stood up and said 'Forget everything I said.' The lawyer that was showing me the office said forget it too. So I waited a while. Then I bought my own building. I had a tough time with those two young doctors. They wanted me run out of town. Finally I said, 'Look, you just leave me alone, and I'll leave you alone. If I'm no good, people will know it. They're not stupid. I won't get any business.' Now I've got as much business as I can handle over there. But there has to be an end to the antagonism. I mean, the patient is supposed to be the important part, caring for the patient."

In the examining rooms he has patients waiting. Two young girls, sisters, get physical exams for a church summer camp. One of the sisters gets a tetanus booster from Ann, while the doctor checks out heart beat, eyes, ears, nose and throat on the other.

In another room, a well-dressed middle-aged woman is coming to have the shingles on her back examined. She still has one large red scaly patch on the middle of her back, but the other areas have faded into slight red marks.

"Well, I'd say another week on this ought to do it, Mrs. Haynes."

"Oh I feel so much better. I thought I was going to go crazy with that itching."

"Let's take a look again next week. Maybe we'll have it licked."

Dr. Grass chuckles on his way back to his office. "You see they tell you now that there is no treatment for shingles. Well, there is one medication that I always had good luck with. They took it off the market a few years back, but I bought up two gallons of the stuff before they did.

"I think the ruination of medicine, the direction it's going, is this specialization. The specialists are meant to be an aid to the general practitioner, not a substitute for him. Nowadays, the definition of a specialist is someone who knows more and more about less and less. The GP is someone who knows less and less about more and more.

"The specialist is a status thing here. I had a woman here in town. She had an infection so she totted herself off to a urologist. He treated her for this urinary infection. And he treated her and treated her. After about six months she came to me and told me all about this treatment. I examined her. She'd had a urinary infection all right, but she had a vaginal infection too. The urologist hadn't looked an inch away from his specialty to see what was causing the problem."

A woman in her thirties is waiting in an examining room.

"You've been feeling dizzy?" he asks. She smiles. "How often?"

"Oh, a few times a day, I think."

"Any nausea, vomiting?" She shakes her head. "You've been doing anything particularly strenuous?"

"No. Just a lot of running around with the kids."

"When was your period?"

"Mmmm, two weeks ago, I guess."

"You're not pregnant? No, let's see, you had . . ."

"Buttonhole operation."

"Right, well, we won't worry about that." He listens to her heart, checks her throat. "You seem OK. Any diarrhea?" She shakes her head. "Problems at home?"

"No, just a lot of running around with the kids."

"I'm going to give you some pills, just enough for a few days, for the dizziness. If it goes beyond that, or if anything else comes up, you let me know."

"Thanks, I will. Goodbye."

"Living in a small community like this, you get involved in things. I've been the county coroner and the county health inspector. Being the coroner, we had some pretty busy times, since I was the only doctor around. The coroner has to pronounce a person dead at the scene of an accident. I remember one time, there was a bad accident out there on the four lane. Truck hit a guy on a tractor. The guy in the truck was dead. The guy on the tractor had his leg ripped open inside his thigh . . . was bleeding real bad. Well, we brought the guy in the tractor right over to the office and started stitching. Meanwhile, the police couldn't move the fellow in the truck until I'd pronounced him dead, and traffic was piled up all over hell. Finally, I got the police to bring the guy over to the office in the ambulance and I walked out here in front of the office and pronounced him dead. First things first. Sometimes you have to twist things a bit to get things done.

"You have to be real careful in a job like that. You think things are cut and dried in a death, but if you take short cuts you can get in trouble. We had a young man, not too long ago, shot himself in his room with a .22. Seemed like a pretty obvious case. But the mother didn't think so. She was sure it had been someone else.

"Oh, we've done a little bit of everything here. Course this is a farm community . . . we have done a few finger amputations here during harvest time. Had one boy run himself through a barbwire fence on a snowmobile. Ripped himself up all around his neck. Well, it was a Sunday. Couldn't get a hold of any of my assistants. So I just did it alone. We do everything here. Hell. I even make house calls occasionally."

There are more patients waiting. An older arthritic woman checking in for more medication. Another older woman with a scabby rash on her swollen legs. She gets more medication for high blood pressure as well. A young mother complaining of diarrhea and nausea. A five-year-old boy getting stitches checked after almost losing a finger in a game with an axe.

"I'm responsible for the nursing home people too. That's fifty more people altogether. But they don't get the attention they should . . . They should have yearly physicals and checkups, but I haven't the time. I'm thinking of hiring another physician's assistant to look after them."

At twelve-thirty Dr. Grass leaves the Randall office in his Cadillac. Ann comes with him to the Center City office for the afternoon. The other two women stay at the Randall office to take calls, and do the paper work and inventory. He leaves Ann off at the second office and goes out to the little hospital at the edge of town.

"Osteopaths are licensed to do everything the medics can do," Dr. Grass says. "In fact, just like the MDs, there is a problem in osteopathy now of too many specialists. They do surgical specialties and the works. In fact, I always like to remember when I get in debates with people, that in the 1950s in California, the state wanted to take over the osteopathic schools. They offered any osteopath who had passed his licensing exam an MD for $50.00. That's a fact."

Dr. Grass leaves his car by the emergency entrance to the hospital. It is dark inside, everything done in glazed yellow brick, with distant overhead lights. His physician's assistant, Fred Hahn, is waiting for him at the nursing station. Fred has already been to see the patients in the hospital once, and goes over the hospital charts with the doctor before they visit them again.

"How is Ellen?" Dr. Grass asked.

"I think she had a pretty rough night. She's still pretty depressed, hasn't been eating very much. But she's alert."

"I've known Ellen since I first moved to this area. People just go on being tough and tough, you know, and you think things are all right. I don't hospitalize people very often for psychiatric problems. But in this case, she's only forty. About a year ago, she lost her husband suddenly. Then a few months later, her mother died. She was remarkable. She seemed to take everything in stride. Then all of a sudden she collapsed, deep depression, couldn't function."

The rooms in the hospital are all equally dark. Ellen, a husky woman with short dark hair and freckles, is in the first bed. She is propped up in bed and smiles warmly when she sees Dr. Grass.

"Hello, dear," he says. "How are things going?"

"I think I'm gonna be all right," she says. "I'm going to get out of this place." She laughs.

"Well, I think we can start cutting down on the medication if you're feeling up to it."

"I have already. They brought pills this morning, but I decided I'd have to start, you know, cutting down so I just didn't take them."

"You don't have to go cold turkey, you know. Think you'll be ready to go home tomorrow?"

"Oh yes. I'm ready." Dr. Grass is sitting next to the bed and she takes his hand and holds it for a few seconds. She is smiling a gruff smile but there are tears in her eyes.

In the next room, a woman in her forties who has been in traction for a week is talking to her husband.

"How's the pain?" the doctor asks.

"Still pretty strong down my right leg."

"Well, I think we'd better send you on up to the big city then," he smiles. "We'll get you set up there with some orthopedic men and see what they can do for you. A week in traction is enough of a test. We'll have to turn you over to someone else. I'll go make a call and let you know when they want you."

There is a doctor's dressing room down the hall. Dr. Grass goes in with Fred to call the orthopedists.

"Yes, Lou. Long distance. Would you get Hingery, Wallace and Arnold at St. Elizabeth's? Whichever one's around. Call me back at the doctor's room. Thanks."

"This woman was injured four years ago," Dr. Grass explains. The phone rings. "Yes, Dr. Arnold. Herb Grass in Randall. I've got a patient I'd like to send up to you." He gives Dr. Arnold the specifics of the case, the history, tests that were given, patient responses. "When would you like to see her? All right . . . Thank you. She'll be there." He turns to Fred. "Would you get her dismissal papers, please, and tell her what the plans are? They'll do a mylogram on her probably. You might explain that to her. I don't know why they didn't do it the last time she was up there."

Dr. Grass and Fred leave the doctor's dressing room and look in on two elderly men recovering from recent heart attacks. Next they visit a middle-aged man with emphysema who asks to be sent home right away.

"I don't know, Ed," Dr. Grass says. "You don't look so good. You still using the oxygen?"

"Not last night," Ed says.

"I thought maybe, since he lives in town, it would be all right," Fred offers cautiously. "Since I'll be at the office all day he can come in easily enough to be checked."

"I suppose. OK. We'll let you go tomorrow, Ed. But I don't want you back here next week."

Once the rounds at the hospital are finished, Fred and Dr. Grass drive to the office in town. There is a full afternoon of patients ahead, then the trip back to Randall for Dr. Grass. A few acute cases will be seen there before going home. There will be phone calls at home, probably, an emergency, possibly.

"There isn't much difference between a DO and a medic," Dr. Grass says. "The medical schools get more money, so their clinical training is a bit better probably. But there isn't much difference.

An osteopath can make as much money as a medic. But I think the osteopath has to work harder for it, has to prove himself all the time. Now, up the next county here, they needed a doctor. These small towns will do anything to get an MD. Up there, I just read in the paper last night, they're building a million dollar clinic and the doctor gets his part rent-free for ten years. Other places give 'em free homes ... who knows what all. You think that would happen to an osteopath? No way."

SUMMARY

DUTIES: *Acts as independent practitioner, similar to an MD, using accepted methods of diagnosis and treatment, including drugs, surgery and psychiatry. The osteopath has special skills in the area of manipulative therapy techniques to correct problems of the muscle and skeletal systems. The emphasis in osteopathy has been in family practice, although specialties can be done as well.*

TRAINING: *The training is similar to that of an MD. Both an MD and an osteopath get an undergraduate degree. The osteopath then takes three to four years of training in a college of osteopathy, plus an internship. For more information, contact:*

American Osteopathic Association
212 East Ohio Street
Chicago, Illinois   60611

SALARY: *$31,000 is an average income after business expenses.*

5

CLINICAL PHARMACIST

"I never worked in a drugstore until my senior year in pharmacy school. Then I found out . . . lick, stick, count and pour. That was it. What a shock."

Steve Connell sits in the staff coffee room before his work day begins. His fingers drum steadily along the sides of a styrofoam cup. His dark eyes peer from behind glasses.

"I drove an ambulance to work my way through college. That was my orientation toward medicine . . . all those crises, all that patient care. The only model I had was a pharmacist in my neighborhood when I was a kid. A great man, and he did a lot of consulting and advising customers. Well, that's pretty much part of the past. The doctors don't consult the pharmacist, the customers don't consult the pharmacist. It's just measuring and typing labels."

For Steve, a change in pharmacist training came along just in time. The doctor of pharmacy, or Pharm D. program, started at the University of California and had made it to the University of Southern California in time for Steve to become part of it. It consists of two years beyond the regular five-year pharmacy program. The extra training comes mostly in clinical settings, working with patients and doctors on proper drug therapy.

"The drug situation is just getting out of hand. No doctor with a reasonably busy practice can keep up with new drugs, new research, even in specialty areas. The clinical pharmacist is an on-the-spot consultant. There may be some initial resistance, but most doctors who have Pharm D.s around find them a great help."

Steve joined the allergy team in this large hospital several years ago. He now works in the child allergy clinic. "There was lots of resistance from the residents and interns in the beginning. But I was hired by the head of the department, Dr. Meyer, which helped a lot. He really wanted me here. Now the new people doing rotations have gotten the idea that I'm here to help them."

Steve finishes his coffee and steps into the corridor of the clinic. Through an open door comes the sound of a nurse putting a child through a lung capacity test.

"Come on now," the nurse cheers. "Push, Jimmy. Push! Push! Push!"

A big plastic schedule board on the wall shows which patients are in which rooms and who is to see them.

"Has Anderson been seen yet?" Steve asks a dark-haired nurse in a red sweater.

"I don't think so. His skin test is done, though."

"OK." With clipboard in hand, Steve heads into one of the examining rooms. "Things can get confusing. We not only have the usual group of residents and interns, but I have a pharmacy student with me as well." Inside the room a thirteen-year-old boy sits on an examining table, his mother in a chair next to him. He isn't wearing a shirt. His long bare arms are spotted with reactions to the skin test given shortly before.

"Robert Anderson?" Steve asks as he steps in. "Hi. And Mrs. Anderson? I'm Steve Connell. I'm a clinical pharmacist and I'd like to get a drug history on Bob if I could?"

Mrs. Anderson smiles.

"Let's see. Bob is thirteen?"

"Yes."

"Pretty stuffy this morning, Bob? Is this your bad time of year?" Bob nods.

"Well, it's always worse this time of year," Mrs. Anderson says. "His eyes get so watery."

Steve turns a page on his clipboard and begins checking answers on a printed form.

"Has Bob ever had side effects from any drug?" Mrs. Anderson shakes her head no. "Allergic or toxic effects from a drug? Has he ever used asthma inhalers, such as Isoproterenol?" She shakes her head again. "How about oral theophylline?" She looks puzzled. "Tedral, Marax . . . those both have theophylline."

"Yes. He's taken Tedral."

"Rectal asthma medications? Injections? Prednisone? Desensitization shots? Has he taken any of the following drugs in the past month: Penicillin? Digitalis? Antacids? Laxatives?"

"I think he took a laxative once," Mrs. Anderson says. "Didn't you, Bob?"

"I don't remember," the boy says.

"Hemorrhoid preparations?" Steve goes on. "Marijuana? Speed? LSD?"

"No. Have you, Bob?" She laughs.

"No," Bob smiles back.

"OK. Thank you, Mrs. Anderson. A doctor will be in shortly to examine Bob. I'll be back with you later in the day to talk about any medications that may be prescribed."

Steve leaves the room and closes the door behind him. His pharmacy student, Allen Simms, is standing outside the door.

"I just *did* a drug history on him," Allen says.

"Oh," Steve looks mildly annoyed. "You mean they sat through the drug history twice and didn't say anything? Damn."

A buzzer goes off on Steve's pocket paging device. He heads down the hall to a hospital phone.

"Steve Connell speaking . . . Oh yes, Dr. Fisher . . . No, I think it was done in 1972 or '73. The results were similar though. I'd be happy to get the paper for you . . . Sure, no problem. Glad you're interested. Thanks for calling."

"Ha!" Steve smiles and makes a note on his clipboard. "That's great. Dr. Fisher is the head of Internal Medicine. Last week I did grand rounds up there. That's a meeting of department staff—doctors, nurses, anyone who's interested. They pick someone to talk about a particular topic. It was the first time a pharmacist had ever done grand rounds in this hospital. Now he's following up on some of the theophylline research. That's one of the major drugs for asthmatics . . . a bronchial dilator. It's used in many different preparations. I got involved in research on theophylline when I worked on the pulmonary ward. They lost a few patients from overdosing. On the basis of work I did then, and later work with Dr. Meyer, we monitor the theophylline blood levels very carefully. The children that are on theophylline therapy either come in or send in blood samples on a regular basis. It's an easily misused drug."

Steve's next patient is another boy, about ten years old. He too, is sitting barechested with the results of the skin tests showing on

CLINICAL PHARMACIST

his arm. His mother hovers nearby. The mother discusses her son's problem with Steve.

"Twice now he's broken out in terrible hives, all over his body. I think it had to be mint Kaopectate. That's the only thing that was different that I can recall. He's taken the regular Kaopectate without any reaction. I know that."

Steve opens the door and calls to one of the allergy nurses.

"Karen, do we have any mint antigen?"

"I don't think so," she says. "I'll check."

"Also," the mother continues, "he wheezes terribly and gets watery eyes after being with the guinea pig at school. The teacher thought he had a cold but every time he has monitor duty and has to clean the guinea pig cage, he comes home a wreck."

"Are you or your husband allergic at all?"

"Yes. We both are." Steve takes notes and then turns to the drug history.

"Anti-coagulants, anticonvulsants, penicillin or sulfa in the last month? . . ." Steve asks. The drug history takes only a short while. Once finished he leaves the room.

On his way to his next patient, Steve stops the allergy nurse in the hall again.

"Mint antigen?" She shakes her head no. "I thought so."

In the next examining room, a young mother and father are with their son and daughter. The boy is about ten, the girl a bit younger. A resident has already begun a physical on the boy, so Steve takes the younger child and the mother into another room to do the drug history.

The mother is an attractive woman. They have come from a neighboring state where they live in a small town. Both the children have been suffering from hay fever.

"Any bad reactions to drugs?" Steve asks, as he reaches the questionnaire.

"Yes. Both Chris and Julie got terrible hives from penicillin. That was when we lived in Chicago."

"Do you have any idea what kind of penicillin it was?"

"No. They were shots."

"We should try to get the records on that if at all possible. Even if it means writing to your doctor in Chicago. Some penicillin injections contain Novocain to slow the absorption. Sometimes people have reactions to the Novocain and then they get written up as having an allergy to penicillin. You don't want to eliminate an important drug like penicillin unless you have to."

"I think I can find out. I'll check. Also Julie, fairly recently, well, she had a cold and the doctor gave her this medicine, tetracycline. Here, I brought the bottle."

"That's a drug that is probably not right for her. It can have some bad side effects. We better contact your doctor and talk this over."

After leaving the room Steve shakes his head. "There's a perfect example. The doctor is out of touch, probably perfectly well intentioned. We don't use tetracycline with children. There are lots of side effects from antibiotics. Some can even cause hearing loss if not used properly."

Dr. Meyer, the head of the child allergy clinic, and an intern are on their way in to examine Julie. Steve confers with Dr. Meyer briefly about Julie's drug history and then leaves.

"You see," Steve explains, "the doctors get their information from the drug detail men, the salesmen who come into the office. Very few companies hire salesmen with any scientific background. The companies have marketing branches and medical branches. It's the marketing branch that makes the final decision about what goes into a drug. Take Tedral, for example. Tedral contains theophylline and ephedrine. Research shows that ephedrine does not add to the effectiveness of the theophylline but increases the side effects, such as nervousness, headaches. But the marketing branch does its research and, because of the trade name or whatever, decides it will continue with the ephedrine. So it stays. Marketing decisions. You can't help but feel a little like a crusader when you see how these critical decisions are being made."

Allen Simms catches Steve before he moves on to his next patient. Allen goes over the drug history he has taken on one of his patients. Part of Steve's job in the clinic is as a teacher. He questions Allen about the particular drug the patient is taking.

"What is the effective blood level for that?" Steve asks. Allen pauses. "You'd better look it up," Steve directs sharply.

In the next room, Mr. and Mrs. Hunt, a couple in their early forties, sit in chairs waiting. Their daughter Angela sits on the examining table in her clothes. She is a beautiful child of twelve, with long blond hair and blue eyes, her cheeks tan from the summer sun. Mrs. Hunt's eyes don't leave the child, even while she speaks to the resident who has already examined Angela.

"When we called in last week they said we could cut the steroids down to every other day. It just didn't work. She loves athletics so much, but two nights ago I picked her up from baseball practice and she could hardly breathe. It was almost as bad as last summer."

"You had a bad time last summer?" the resident asks.

"I picked her up at the swimming pool one night," Mrs. Hunt says. "And I had to give her an adrenalin injection right there in the parking lot. That was the worst, but she had lots of bad nights. It eased off some during the winter, but now . . . I don't know."

"Does the Aminophyllin get her through the night?"

"Well, she's supposed to take that every four hours. I usually wake her at eleven, before I go to bed. But when I don't wake her again until I get up at six. By that time she's usually pretty wheezy."

"Is she taking the Prednisone, the steroids, now?" Steve asks.

"Well, we called in yesterday and whoever we talked to said to go back to every day again."

"How long has it been now, two weeks on daily steroids?" Steve asks, looking over Angela's chart.

"A bit more than that."

"The steroids are clearly effective," Steve says. "But we don't like to leave children on them for long periods of time. It's possible to stunt their growth with extended use. Of course she has no danger signs now at all."

"She's using an inhaler too?" the resident asks.

"Yes, she uses the inhaler too, for the sudden attacks."

"You have quite a pack to take to school with you, don't you, Angela?" Steve smiles. The child smiles and nods.

"It's a little embarrassing for her at school," Mrs. Hunt says. "Sometimes she gets home from school wheezing because she's put off taking her medication."

"That can be hard." Steve steps into the hall and catches Dr. Meyer. "Dr. Meyer. Could you spend a minute with the Hunts?"

"How do you do?" Dr. Meyer steps in and closes the door behind him. "Angela, are you still having problems?"

"It's better than last summer, but still pretty bad," Mr. Hunt says.

"Dr. Meyer, I'm wondering about that new steroid inhaler, the experimental one," Steve says, "Wouldn't that get the ingredient down to the lungs and maybe be less risky than the oral doses? She's been on Prednisone for two weeks now." Dr. Meyer takes Angela's record from Steve and looks it over quickly.

"I think that would be a good thing to try. We'll cut down the oral Prednisone, but not cut it out altogether yet. Since they're from out of town, you'd better give them one of our samples in the supply room. They won't be able to get them in their drugstore yet. Did you have a blood sample drawn, Angela?"

"Yes."

"We'll want to check the theophylline level. We might be able to raise that a bit yet. Let's see if we can't get these symptoms under control." Dr. Meyer leaves and the resident gets the new inhaler from the drug supply room.

"OK, Angela," Steve moves his chair over so he is sitting next to Angela. "I'm going to show you how to use this. It's very important that you use it right so it can help. Now, you take the plastic cap off and here is where the mist will come out. Squeeze the top here... see, it's like your other inhaler. Now I want you to blow out for three counts and then on four, you inhale deeply. Like this, one... two... three... in! OK. Let's have you try."

Angela takes the inhaler and self-consciously blows out, then in.

"I don't think she got it," the resident says.

"Let's try it again. One... two... three... in! OK, she got it that time. Don't you think she did?" He turns to Mr. Hunt.

"Yeah. Her eyes crossed," Mr. Hunt laughs.

"It tastes a little funny," Angela says.

"OK. You folks might as well go get some lunch," Steve says. "The blood tests should be done by the time you get back and we'll meet with you around one o'clock. I'm going to make a list of Angela's medications and the timing of them so you will have it all spelled out." Mrs. Hunt opens her pocketbook to show them all the bottles she carries with her. "Yes, I know. It's a lot. You've all done a great job. Angela, I'm very proud of you. I know this is tough on you, especially in the summer, having your sports cut down and all. But you've done a fine job..." Angela bites her lip and then the tears start rolling down her cheek. Then the tears are rolling down her mother's cheek, and her father, smiling, wipes his eyes behind his glasses. "That's good," Steve says. "That's just fine. You all needed that."

After finishing with the Hunts, Steve and the resident walk together to a noon conference with the clinic staff.

"I don't know," the resident says. "Every time the Hunts call in someone gives the kid another blast of steroids. It can't go on forever."

"I don't think she's been mismanaged," Steve says. "After all, the kid has severe attacks. It may be a choice between the steroids or the hospital."

The conference is in a small room with a large table and folding chairs around it. Dr. Meyer attends, as do the two allergy nurses, two residents, a medical student and two pharmacy students.

"Jeff," Dr. Meyer says, addressing one of the pharmacy students. "You were going to discuss Metaproterenol for us."

Jeff reads a brief paper to the group on the drug, its effects and side effects. "Actually," he concludes, "I can't understand why the FDA passed it. There are already several drugs on the market with higher effectiveness."

"The FDA will pass it," Dr. Meyer says, "if it is not toxic and effects the condition it is meant to effect. It doesn't have to be the most effective, it just has to have some effect on a given condition. I did have a case recently where Metaproterenol knocked out a final annoying symptom for a patient who had already been treated dramatically with other drugs."

One of the residents presents a paper on the seventy-year history of desensitization shots, which began with a doctor putting serum from flowers in the eyes of his patients.

"The mechanism for protection is still unknown. That is, there is still little concrete data to show which patients can be helped by desensitization and which cannot," the resident concludes.

"This is an area," Dr. Meyer says, "where basic research is badly needed. The clinical research cannot do the trick. You have to round up allergic patients in a given area and by the time you match them for treatment groups you don't have enough numbers to be significant. With chronic asthmatics, people who have symptoms all year, my own experience tells me the shots are not very effective. If you have a patient with a heavy hay fever component and more seasonal asthma, you have a better chance. But we're faced with a clinical situation where we have to work from inadequate data. How do you make a decision for a patient to go through the nuisance of shots? I don't know."

"How about other desensitization therapies, like poison ivy?"

"I read recently that the capsule poison ivy desensitizer caused rectal poison ivy," Steve offers with a smile.

"My own feeling about the poison ivy desensitization is that it's a waste," Dr. Meyer says. "Unless a person is a professional gardener or something, he can learn to stay away from it."

"I agree," Steve says. "Plus, for those people who get bad cases from accidental exposure, it only takes a short course with steroids to clear it up."

With the noon conference over, the rest of Steve's day is spent meeting again with the patients he saw in the morning. Steve carefully describes the different medications that have been prescribed and makes up a sheet for each patient showing the dosage and times. He describes the effect the drugs should have, and how to look for bad reactions.

"I wouldn't want to spend every day like this," Steve says as he gets ready to leave. "I'm really just here in the clinic two or three days a week. The research and teaching break things up for me. I put a lot into the patients. I really feel I give them my best. A doctor who has to see patients all the time can get burned out.

"I do regret sometimes that I didn't get into medical school. I grew up with the idea that I was going to be a doctor. My mother, I guess. It can be frustrating, only being able to take care of the patients so far. On the other hand, I have a chance to be a pace setter. I feel like I'm influencing not just the patients but the professional people around me.

"I don't know how long I'll stay in this setting. Clinical pharmacists are beginning to be in demand. I have a friend who is in practice with several doctors and he gets a percentage of their gross. He rakes in a lot of money. For me, now, it's a matter of choosing between the intellectual and the financial rewards. The financial ones might look good some day. But, for now, I'm content."

SUMMARY

DUTIES: *Uses specific knowledge of drugs in clinical teamwork. Assists physicians in the prescription of drugs and advises and edu-*

cates patients in the proper use of drugs. Works in hospital teams or in group practice with private physicians.

TRAINING: *The usual training for a licensed pharmacist is a five-year school of pharmacy after high-school graduation. The clinical pharmacist or doctor of pharmacy degree is a six-year program, the sixth year made up mostly of clinical work. For more information, contact:*

> *American Association of Colleges of Pharmacy*
> *4630 Montgomery Avenue, Suite 201*
> *Bethesda, Maryland   20014*

SALARY: *$13,000–22,000.*

6

NURSE MIDWIFE

"I worked six years in obstetrics after I got my RN. It was fun, but I felt frustrated. I only saw the mothers for a couple of days while they were hospitalized. When they left, I'd lose touch. Now, as a certified nurse midwife, I can follow them for almost a year. It's much more satisfying for both of us."

Evelyn Francis reminisces as her car leaves the expressway and eases into the slower traffic past a shopping mall. She has short brown hair and wears a solid green dress. Her manner is calm, and low keyed.

Evelyn was lucky. Her excellent background in obstetrics earned her quick acceptance into the Nurse-Midwife Program at the State University of New York's College of Health Related Professions in Brooklyn. Most of the American programs now have long waiting lists and many American nurses have gone abroad to get their midwifery education.

"I didn't want to go to Kentucky to the Frontier Nursing Service Midwife program. Rural life is just not for me. I can't imagine myself driving a jeep." She laughs. "I didn't want to go to England either."

The midwifery course was flexible. Since she was an experienced nurse in obstetrics, she concentrated on learning how to make medical decisions about patient care all through pregnancy. After finishing the school year, there was a comprehensive national exam to pass. Most states will license midwives who pass the exam, although there are differences in how much they will allow midwives to do. Forty-eight states now have licensure laws that allow nurse midwives to participate in at least part of the maternity care for patients. Massachusetts and Colorado have just passed laws allowing nurse midwives to do everything, including deliveries. It took seven years to get the law passed in Massachusetts.

"It's been a struggle to gain acceptance. Parents have been an important source of pressure to change the laws. Some physicians are very hostile. Others are supportive. They recognize and appreciate the way we complement each other in our services to the parents."

After passing the national exam, a nurse midwife can choose to go through an internship or go directly into practice.

"For some people, an internship is a good idea," Evelyn explains. "You need some time to develop confidence in making patient-management decisions. The close supervision can be a great help with this." Evelyn turns into the driveway of the Salvation Army's Booth Maternity Center. It is an inconspicuous, three-story yellow brick building set well back from the street. That inconspicuous building, however, has served as a seed-bed for a revolution in patient care.

Seven years ago, Booth Memorial, as it was called then, was a building that had almost outlived its purpose. The Salvation Army had built Booth as a place for unwed mothers to have their babies in privacy. Middle- and upper-class families would send their teenage daughters there to have their illegitimate babies and avoid scandal. Times, however, changed. Abortions and contraceptives became more readily available. There wasn't the same stigma attached to being a single parent. As a result, fewer and fewer women were coming to Booth. The building was almost empty.

Three people involved in providing obstetrical care came to Booth with a plan. They were looking for a place where obstetric rules could be relaxed, where care could be more family-centered and where, most of all, parents could make most of the decisions about how their baby was to be delivered. After many months of planning and preparation, Booth Memorial became Booth Maternity Center. The program started with one physician and three midwives. They averaged about 20 deliveries a month during the first year. Now they average 120 deliveries a month and have three physicians and ten nurse midwives on the staff. There isn't room for all the people who want their babies delivered at Booth.

The receptionist waves at Evelyn as she comes in the door.

"She had a little girl," Evelyn says.

"Oh that's wonderful. Her grandmother will be very happy. Did you deliver?"

"No, I circulated," Evelyn says.

Evelyn takes the elevator to the second floor. She wants to check on several of the patients before the office hours start. She likes the 8:00 a.m. to 4:00 p.m. shift. More variety. She checks the chart on a baby sleeping in the nursery, then walks to the room across the hall.

"Hi, Virginia, how are you doing?" Evelyn asks.

"Fine, a little tired," Virginia says.

"I peeked at your baby in the nursery. He's beautiful. Everything's fine. Did Dr. Wilson talk to you about his examination?" Virginia nods.

Evelyn leaves Virginia and walks down the corridor toward the desk. There are only five double-occupancy patient rooms on the floor, small by most hospital standards. The labor and delivery suite is right next to the patient rooms. In many hospitals they are located on a separate floor.

"A small place like this helps all the mothers understand what is going on, and they can participate in it. When it's busy they know why, and who it is. They don't get upset if we can't get to them right at the minute they want us. Everybody shares in the excitement."

She walks through the swinging doors that separate the labor and delivery rooms from the patient floor. The labor room she enters is dimly lit and quiet. There are cloth color prints on the wall. A young woman is lying on her right side. One of the midwives is acting as the main support person. She is leaning close to her, stroking her head and handing her ice chips. The woman's face is white, her lips are trembling. Her mother, dressed in a blue surgical suit, stands massaging her feet. The water bag that surrounds the fetus during its nine months has been broken and a lead from a fetal monitor has been inserted and attached to the scalp of the fetus. The beeps on the monitor are regular. Alice, the nurse midwife who has been assisting, stops massaging the woman's abdomen and looks at the paper printout from the monitor.

"Everything's fine. That was a big contraction, Martha." Alice says.

The monitor charts the heart beat of the baby and the mother's contractions. They are watching to make sure that beats do not continue to slow after the contraction. That could mean problems. The placenta might not be pushing through the supply of oxygen and nutrients that the fetus needs. The beats, however, have returned to normal after the contraction.

"How are you doing, Miriam?" Evelyn asks.

Martha's mother shrugs and smiles.

"It's been eight hours and Martha's cervix has dilated to seven centimeters. Her contractions are coming about two minutes apart. It will be a while yet. Miriam, why don't you go down and get some coffee? Diane will take over for you," Alice says.

Diane, a nurse who has just entered the room, smiles and takes Miriam's place. Miriam squeezes Martha's hand and starts to leave.

"Get some breakfast in you too, Miriam," Evelyn says.

Martha, according to their graphs, has not progressed rapidly enough, and the baby is still high in the pelvic area. That's a signal to call in one of the physicians on the staff for a consultation. He will probably order an X ray to determine if the mother's pelvic bones are too small to allow the baby to come through. A Caesarean delivery may be required. The doctor and the midwife will discuss the X ray results together and decide.

Across the hall, in the other labor room, Mary's labor seems to be going according to schedule. Her husband, George, is her support person. He is coaching her with her breathing during contractions. Barbara, the midwife, is massaging her abdomen. Evelyn observes for a few minutes then heads downstairs. Barbara will be off that afternoon. She will probably be filling in for the last few hours of the labor.

"We don't carry a specific case load of parents. We're just too big for that," Evelyn explains. "We're all part of the same team at Booth and we take turns seeing patients during their prenatal visits. If the parents want a specific midwife, we try to arrange it. But they generally understand that all of us are interested in their care and that it may be difficult to see the same midwife at each visit."

It is a few minutes before the office hours start and Evelyn wants to follow up on three patients she saw the day before. She pulls out the three records and leafs through them. The B scan, or sonogram, a picture similar to an X ray but made with sound waves, for Mrs. Wilson's fetus, has been scheduled for Friday. She will call her later to let her know. This is going to be her third Caesarean section and they need to make sure of the date. The B scan will help pinpoint it.

Another patient is of special concern to Evelyn. She spent most of her time in the clinic session sobbing. She's alone. She moved from Maine to have her baby at Booth. She can't get work. Evelyn wanted to make sure that an appointment with the social worker had been scheduled.

"It's very helpful to have the social workers. I remember several weeks ago I got a call. The woman told me her name, told me she had had her baby at Booth four weeks ago and that she was going to kill herself. We got her record, found out she had been seeing one of the social workers, and talked her into coming in for a visit."

The last woman whose chart Evelyn pulls was told yesterday that her fetus was dead.

"I talked to her late in the day by phone. She said she was putting the baby clothes away and that's a good sign. Most can't bring themselves to do that. I want to make sure she gets an appointment with the social worker too. She needs plenty of support right now."

The office area has begun to fill up. There are women in various stages of pregnancy, babies, and fathers sitting in the chairs that line the hall. Two one-year-olds totter unsteadily down the hall. Several mothers are displaying their babies to each other. The mood is festive, chaotic. In the glass case at the entrance T-shirts are displayed for sale. One reads: Booth Maternity Center: Labor Coach.

The wall is lined with photographs and paintings of pregnant women and of fathers and mothers with their infants. The pictures were donated by former patients, sometimes in lieu of payments. The whole cost for Booth's service to patients, the before and after visits and the hospitalization, is about $1,200.

"Some people just asume that because most of the care is given by midwives it will cost a lot less. We get a little irritated by that. The overall cost is about the same as elsewhere in this area, but we feel we're giving the patient a lot more time and attention for their money."

"Hi . . . There's one of my deliveries," Evelyn says.

"Yup, plucked with your very own hands," says a woman seated next to the counter with the charts. She smiles and hands Evelyn a two-month-old baby girl. Their conversation is interrupted by another midwife who has the woman's chart and beckons her into one of the examination rooms.

Evelyn picks up another chart from the top of the pile. The chart keeps a record of all of the contacts with the patient. Notes are made on the preference of the mother, the kind of medication for labor, if she wants any, who her support person or persons are, and what kind of childbirth education classes she's taking. The classes aren't required but all patients are urged to get into one. Weight, blood pressure and the results of urine tests are entered after each visit. Blood tests are taken routinely every three months and also entered into the record. The midwife makes notes in the chart after each visit, evaluating the patient and indicating what actions are planned in caring for the patient.

Evelyn enters an examining room. A woman is sitting on the examining table. Her husband sits next to her. He has a tape recorder with him. The woman has a pad and a pencil.

"Hi. You wanted to see a midwife today?"

The woman nods. "I've seen two of the doctors and I'd like to meet more of the midwives."

"Do you want to ask your questions first?"

"Who checks the baby after she or he is born?" the woman asks, looking at the notes on her pad.

"The midwife does a quick check to see if the baby is breathing well and if all limbs are intact. A neonatologist from Jefferson Medical School does a more detailed examination every day. The neonatologist is a doctor who specializes in the care of newborn babies."

"Will I be told if something is wrong?"

"Yes. We share everything with you."

"If everything is OK, will the doctor still stop by and tell me?"

"Oh yes."

"My leg tends to go to sleep."

Evelyn explains some exercises that will help relieve the pressure of the uterus that is causing the problem.

"We live two and a half hours from here. Is that going to be a problem?" the woman asks.

"Well, some people come here from as far away as New York. A lot depends on how big the baby is. The bigger the baby the slower you'll have to drive. Some people have even come to the city to stay during the last week."

"How about circumcision?"

"You'll have to ask for it. The doctors here don't feel it's necessary anymore. It's like tonsillectomies. They don't do them as often now. Anyway, it's not a decision you have to make right now."

"Yeah, we have to see if it's a boy first," the husband says.

They all laugh.

"Have you signed up for classes yet?" Evelyn asks.

The woman shakes her head.

"Well, you should before you leave today. Of course, you could take a class nearer where you live. It would be more convenient."

"Oh no, we'd like to get to know the people here," she says.

"The last session of the course here is about how to have a baby in an automobile. It rarely happens, but knowing what to do keeps people from getting panicky."

Both the husband and wife laugh nervously.

Evelyn begins the examination. She shares the lab results with them. Everything is normal. She measures the growth of the uterus with a tape from the pubic bone to the top of the uterus.

"You grew seven centimeters. What happened?" she asks.

"Big holiday weekend," the husband says, smiling.

"Well, we don't scold people here. Your weight is OK and the other tests are normal. We'll just dismiss it as a splurge."

They pause while the woman writes down all the results and measurements recorded on the folder into her notebook. Evelyn takes out the doptone, a device for listening to the heartbeat of the fetus. The husband starts his tape recorder. They listen to the swishing sound of the placental beat and then Evelyn locates the louder, more distinct beats of the fetus.

"Is it good?"

"Oh, yes, fine."

"Will we be able to bring the tape recorder into the delivery room? Of course, I insist on the right to remove any sections of the recording I don't like," the woman smiles.

"Oh, yes, you can bring anything you like. If you bring a camera, try to bring a simple one so that we can operate it too. OK, everything is fine. We'll see you again in four weeks."

Jenny, Evelyn's next patient, has brought her baby with her. While a friend holds the baby, Evelyn checks Jenny to see that the pelvic organs have returned to normal following the baby's birth. They discuss the various choices in terms of contraception and Jenny settles on the IUD.

The morning passes quickly. A woman in the last month of pregnancy comes in with swelling in her legs. Evelyn prescribes rest on her left side for twenty minutes and several quarts of water each day.

"It works. We're getting back to more natural methods now. We used to use diuretics, drugs that get out the excess water in the body tissue, but there are side effects both on the mother and the baby."

Another woman is interested in a Leboyer bath. Her husband is excited about it. Leboyer, a French doctor, advocates darkened surroundings and a gentle bath in a glass tub for the newborn. Evelyn explains Booth's ideas about the bath. She points out the problems with getting the water temperature and pressure just right. Also, the midwives like to give the baby right to the mother and get her involved right away. That closeness, they feel, is more important than the bath.

On her way to the cafeteria Evelyn passes a couple with a baby. The baby has a rash. The man has a cast on his arm. Evelyn asks about the rash and the husband's cast and then heads for the stairs.

"It always seems that nurses and doctors have the most problems in delivery," Evelyn laughs. "She's a nurse. She had fifteen hours of prelabor contractions before her cervix began to change, and her labor lasted many hours. Her husband had a slight bone fracture from falling down that he didn't know about. Toward the end, when he was helping her push, his arm broke."

Three midwives who have just come to Booth for the refresher course join Evelyn at lunch. Booth offers a program for midwives trained overseas to help them prepare for the national exams. Two had their midwifery training in England, one in Australia. It is much easier to get into the programs there, not the same backlog as in the United States. They are excited about the amount of participation Booth provides the parents.

"It's all changing so quickly," Evelyn says. "When I started working on an obstetric unit in 1963 it was so different. All the mothers were knocked out. We used large doses of Demerol and Phenergan and on top of that, scopolamine. Scopolamine creates amnesia, so the mothers can't remember what happened afterwards. It also has a very disorienting effect. I can remember one time when we were very busy, I caught a woman crawling out of a delivery room on her hands and knees. She said she had to go to the bathroom. She delivered a few minutes later. It was crazy. I got a lot of experience with obstetrics though. We would do everything for the mothers and the doctors would arrive just in time to catch the baby. Sometimes they didn't get there in time."

"Some women want to be knocked out," said one of the midwives taking the refresher course, recalling her experiences in England.

"Sure, but they should have a choice," Evelyn says.

The others nod in agreement.

After her lunch Evelyn checks back on the obstetric floor. The X rays on Martha had shown that the bones of the pelvis were not wide enough for a normal delivery. A Caesarean section was performed. Martha was awake and saw the baby as it was born. A regional block anesthetic was used so there was no pain. Her mother acted as support person. Dr. Nelson performed the operation and Alice, the other midwife on duty, assisted. The baby girl is now asleep in the nursery.

"Hi, Martha. Congratulations. Let me get a bag of ice for you to put on the stitches. It will make you a little more comfortable."

Martha's face is white, her eyes are red, but she manages a smile.

"There, there, baby, you did fine," her mother says.

Eighty percent of the babies born at Booth are delivered by midwives. The more complicated deliveries that require forceps or a Caesarean section are performed by the physicians.

Evelyn enters one of the delivery rooms.

"Hi, Mary, Hi, George, remember me?" Evelyn says.

George nods.

"Evelyn is going to take over now," Barbara says. "Everything is going fine. Contractions are about a minute or two apart, the cervix is almost fully dilated."

The room is dimly lit. Mary is in a semi-reclining position. She can help push better in this position when the baby starts coming.

George wipes her forehead.

"Come on, Mary, concentrate on the breathing. Hout Hout, Whew," he says.

Mary mimics him. She squirms.

"Oh, ow, it hurts too much!" Mary's eyes dart around the room. "Water," she says.

"Come on, Mary, you can do it," Evelyn says.

If Mary was not so far along in her labor, Evelyn would suggest an injection of Demerol to take the edge off the pain. She knows, however, that Mary wants to have the baby without medication, and she'll be able to with just a little encouragement.

George wipes her face with a cold washrag. She is sweating. George begins to rub the inside of her legs. She is fully dilated now. The pushing begins.

"Ugh." Mary's face turns red.

"Take it easy, Mary. There is no hurry. Relax between the pushes," Evelyn says, touching her shoulder.

It is almost an hour before the top of the baby's head is at the opening of the birth canal. Evelyn checks the size of the opening. She will need to cut a wider opening to prevent tearing.

"It's a tight fit, Mary. Looks like an episiotomy would be a good idea."

Mary nods her consent.

Evelyn injects a local anesthetic into the tissue and makes the incision.

"OK, Mary, the head's coming, push just a little."

George stands behind her helping to raise her body to push.

"Ugh."

"Uh, huh. Uh, huh," George and Mary pant in unison.

"OK, Mary, the head's out. Give another push."

Mary groans.

"Here it is, hey, you have a son," Evelyn calls from behind her surgical mask.

Evelyn continues to suck the mucus out from the mouth and nose of the glistening infant with a bulb syringe. She holds him to her chest and gently rubs his back. The nurse hands her a cloth to wipe his face. The baby is breathing, uttering a few whimpers. Evelyn continues to massage him.

"Ah, he's just fine, Mary."

"Hold it. I got to get a picture," George says.

"Take the lens cap off, George," Evelyn says.

Evelyn places the baby on Mary's stomach, and places a blanket over both of them. Mary is giggling.

"Hi, there, little George, you going to smile for me? Oh, you're precious!" Mary exclaims.

The baby begins to feed at her breast. George snaps some more pictures.

The placenta comes out painlessly a few minutes later. Evelyn clamps and cuts the umbilical cord. She then checks the vaginal opening for tears and begins to sew up the episiotomy.

George now takes the baby.

"Don't worry, George, he's not that fragile," Evelyn says.

George relaxes a little bit. He smiles.

"Hey, some ballplayer, huh?" he says.

By the time Mary is back in her room, she's almost asleep. George is showing the baby off to some of the nurses at the nursing station.

Evelyn completes Mary's chart, checks on her one more time, then changes her clothes to go home.

SUMMARY

DUTIES: *As part of the obstetrical team, the nurse midwife cares for the expectant mother before, during and after birth. The midwife does the routine regular checkups, takes blood pressure, weight and pelvic measurements. S/he will answer questions from the patient and educate the prospective parents about delivery procedures and pre- and post-natal care. S/he will usually be present during the delivery, which may or may not be attended by a physician. The degree of independence the midwife has varies greatly from state to state. In some states, the midwife is allowed to deliver babies in consultation with a physician, but without his/her presence.*

TRAINING: *The special midwife training comes after the RN degree. The RN degree can come from a two-year associate arts degree, a three-year hospital program or a four-year BA. The midwife's training is usually eight months beyond the RN. A master's degree in midwifery is twelve to twenty-four months in addition to the BA. For more information, contact:*

> *American College of Nurse Midwives*
> *1000 Vermont Avenue NW, Suite 5000*
> *Washington, D.C. 20005*

SALARY: *Starts at $10,000–12,000.*

RELATED OCCUPATIONS

OPTOMETRIST

DUTIES: *The optometrist examines eyes for vision problems. S/he can prescribe, prepare and fit glasses and contact lenses. If evidence of eye disease is present, the optometrist will refer the client to an ophthalmologist, a physician whose specialty is the eye.*

TRAINING: *The optometrist needs two years of college and then enters a four-year course of professional training in optometry. For more information, contact:*

> *American Optometric Association*
> *7000 Chippewa Street*
> *St. Louis, Missouri   63119*

SALARY: *$15,500 to start. In private practice, an optometrist can earn above $30,000.*

PODIATRIST

DUTIES: *The podiatrist diagnoses and treats foot diseases and deformities. S/he may perform surgery, fit corrective devices, take X rays and do blood tests. Podiatrists treat bunions, calluses, ingrown toenails and arch disabilities. Podiatrists refer patients to physicians if there are any signs of abnormalities other than foot problems.*

TRAINING: *There are currently six colleges of podiatry in this country. Two years of regular college are required before entering a school of podiatry. The training is two years at a school of podiatry and two years of clinical work. For more information, contact:*

> *American Association of Colleges of Podiatric Medicine*
> *20 Chevy Chase Circle NW*
> *Washington, D.C.   20015*

SALARY: *$42,000 is the average income.*

PATHOLOGIST

DUTIES: *The pathologist is a physician with a specialty in the diagnosis of disease. There are two kinds of pathologists. The clinical pathologist makes diagnoses from tests run at hospitals and clinics. These include blood tests, pap smears and other laboratory tests.*

Anatomic pathologists make diagnoses from examining parts of the body. The pathologist in a hospital is in charge of all the laboratory tests. An anatomic pathologist is responsible for all the autopsies at her/his place of work. The pathologist has very little patient contact. S/he works largely in the laboratory setting.

TRAINING: *The training period is long. Four years of undergraduate school, three years of medical school and at least a four-year residency in pathology. For more information, contact:*

> American Society for Clinical Pathology
> 2100 West Harrison
> Chicago, Illinois 60612

SALARY: *Salaries vary greatly. The physician is the highest paid professional in the country, and the pathologist is a highly paid physician. Income for physicians averages around $54,000.*

MEDICAL SOCIAL WORKER

DUTIES: *Medical social workers must understand the problems of people who are ill or disabled. They work to move patients out of the hospital and back to their homes. They act as an advocate and go-between for the patient in dealings with various social agencies in the community, such as food programs and visiting nurses. Medical social workers are employed in hospitals, clinics and public and private health departments.*

TRAINING: *A degree in social work from a four-year college is required. For more information, contact:*

> National Association of Social Workers
> 15 and H Street NW
> 600 Southern Building
> Washington, D.C. 20005

SALARY: *$8,000 to start. May go as high as $15,000.*

DENTIST

DUTIES: *The dentist treats ailments of the gums and teeth. S/he fills cavities, extracts teeth and provides dentures. Specialty areas include oral surgery and orthodontia, or braces.*

TRAINING: *A person must have at least two years of college before entering dental school. The dental school training is a four-year course. Two more years are needed for a specialty area. For more information, contact:*

> American Dental Association
> 211 East Chicago Avenue
> Chicago, Illinois   60611

SALARY: *$15,000 to start. Average income is around $38,000.*

VETERINARIAN

DUTIES: *The veterinarian takes care of the health problems of animals and is also a figure in disease prevention among humans. In treatment of animals, the veterinarian uses many of the technological advances used in human medicine, including surgery, X rays and drugs. Specialty areas, such as surgery, are also developing in veterinary medicine.*

TRAINING: *A person must have two years of college before starting veterinary school. The college of veterinary medicine is a four-year program. There are only nineteen veterinary colleges in the country, so competition for acceptance can be surprisingly tough. For more information, contact:*

> American Veterinary Medicine Association
> 930 North Meacham Road
> Schaumburg, Illinois   60172

SALARY: *$13,000 to start. Private practice salaries vary greatly, but average around $35,000.*

LICENSED PRACTICAL NURSE

DUTIES: *The LPN works under the direction of a physician or a registered nurse, providing routine care. This may include collecting specimens, dressing wounds, giving enemas, taking temperatures and blood pressures. Duties vary, depending on how specialized the registered nurses are. LPNs can regulate IV bottles and do much of the RN's work.*

TRAINING: *The LPN training programs are usually one year in a vocational-technical school or community college. At least two years of high school are required for the training program. For more information, contact:*

*National Association for Practical Nurse Education and Service
122 East 42nd Street
New York, New York 10017*

SALARY: *$7,500 is the average starting salary.*

HEALTH PHYSICIST

DUTIES: *Because of the increased use of radiation in treatment and diagnosis of disease, the medical field is bringing in special physicists to cope with the hazards. Health physicists were established as a group in 1942 to look after the health of nuclear workers and the public at large. They are involved in research, consulting and enforcement of regulations. They work at federal agencies, hospitals and nuclear power plants.*

TRAINING: *Many university physics departments offer MS and Ph.D degrees in Health Physics, after the regular four years of college. There are also positions available as health physics technicians to assist the health physicist. These positions require two years of college. For more information, contact:*

*Health Physics Society
P.O. Box 156
East Weymouth, Massachusetts 02189*

SALARY: *$8,550–25,000, depending on education.*

BIOMEDICAL ENGINEER

DUTIES: *Biomedical engineers are used to solve medical and health-related problems that have engineering components. Some work on the development of artificial hearts and kidneys, lasers and pacemakers. Others adapt computers to hospital systems to increase efficiency. They may work in medical settings or in private medically-related industries.*

TRAINING: *Entrance level for the biomedical engineer requires a BS. MS or Ph.D degrees are desirable. For more information, contact:*

*Alliance for Engineering in Medicine and Biology
3900 Wisconsin Avenue, NW, Suite 300
Washington, D.C. 20016*

SALARY: *$14,000–21,000 to start, depending on education.*

CHIROPRACTOR

DUTIES: *The chiropractor believes that the nervous system is central to the general health of the individual. If the nervous system is interfered with, the resistance of the body to disease is weakened. The chiropractor uses manipulation of the body, especially the spine, to improve health and relieve pain. S/he may use X rays and water, heat, light, diet and exercise therapy in her/his treatment of patients.*

TRAINING: *The chiropractor must have two years of college before entering chiropractic school. Chiropractic school takes four years. There are about twelve chiropractic schools in the country now, but they are increasing. For more information, contact:*

>American Chiropractic Association
>2200 Grand Avenue
>Des Moines, Iowa   50312

SALARY: *$12,000–15,000 to start. Salaries may rise to $28,000.*

MEDICAL ILLUSTRATOR

DUTIES: *The medical illustrator makes drawings and models of medical and surgical findings for teaching, publishing or research. S/he may do drawings for presentations or for use in textbooks. S/he meets with scientists to determine their needs. S/he may assist in the overall styling of medical books.*

TRAINING: *The medical illustrator needs three to four years of college with emphasis on biology, zoology and anatomy. Then s/he must take two years of training in a school of medical illustration. For more information, contact:*

>The Association of Medical Illustrators
>738 Keystone Avenue
>River Forest, Illinois   60305

SALARY: *$13,000–15,000 to start.*

EMBALMER

DUTIES: *The embalmer prepares the dead body for burial in conformity with state health laws. S/he may need to restore a dis-*

figured face, dress the body for the funeral and place it in the casket. Most embalmers work in funeral homes, but there are some positions in hospitals.

TRAINING: *The state requirements that an embalmer must meet vary. Embalming may involve an apprenticeship-traineeship of one to two years, or it may involve a two- to three-year course leading to a BS in funeral service education. For more information, contact:*

> *American Board of Funeral Service Education*
> *201 Columbus Street*
> *Fairmont, West Virginia   26554*

SALARY: *$9,000–10,000 to start.*

FAMILY PRACTICE PHYSICIAN

DUTIES: *The family practice physician is a recently recognized specialty and now has its own board exam for the specialty. It was created to offset the influence of specialization among physicians. The family practice physician attempts to deal with the general health of the family in a community. S/he is specially trained in pediatrics, psychiatry, surgery and obstetrics. Depending on the medical community s/he works in, s/he may chose not to do surgery or obstetrics. The family practice physician tends to work in a group practice and, more than other MDs, attempts to work in areas where there is a shortage of primary care physicians.*

TRAINING: *The family practice physician has a three-year specialty training after the three years of medical school. For more information, contact:*

> *The American Academy of Family Physicians*
> *1740 West 92 Street*
> *Kansas City, Missouri   64114*

SALARY: *Specific figures for the family physician are not available. The average income for physicians in general is $54,000.*

DIALYSIS TECHNICIAN

DUTIES: *The dialysis technician sets up and operates the kidney machine for people who need the periodic dialysis treatment to stay alive. This involves assembling the machine, mixing the solutions needed and transporting the patient. The dialysis technician takes the blood pressure, respiratory rate and pulse and the blood samples needed. The dialysis technician is present during the treatment, making sure the solution is right, and giving oxygen and blood as needed. S/he is also in charge of maintaining the machine, ordering supplies and cleaning up.*

TRAINING: *The dialysis technician must have an RN degree, and then takes one to three months of training under the supervision of a physician. For more information, contact:*

> *American Nursing Association*
> *10 Columbus Circle*
> *New York, New York 10019*

SALARY: *Salary ranges are similar to those for an RN. Salaries start around $11,500.*

therapists and technicians

It is in the area of therapists and technicians that the influence of modern medical technology has been most visible. The jobs of laboratory technologist and respiratory therapist, for example, are directly connected to the creation of new machinery and diagnostic tools. This is also apparent in many of the other occupations discussed in this section. In "Related Occupations," you will read about the EEG technician, the nuclear medical technologist and the cytotechnologist. These are all personnel trained to use the new machines of modern medicine.

The title "therapist," while it is sometimes applied to highly technical medicine, reflects more of a mixture of old and new techniques. The clinical psychologist, while well-schooled in modern techniques, may be using nineteenth century psychology along with the latest therapy.

It should be noted that many of the therapy and technician jobs have different levels, depending on the degree of education acquired. Along with the laboratory technologist, for example, there are also laboratory technicians, who need less training, and laboratory aides, who often work with just on-the-job training. In the area of mental health, there are psychiatric technicians and psychiatric aides who assist the psychiatrist and psychologist in their work. There are physical therapists, physical therapy technicians and physical therapy assistants. These levels should be kept in mind as alternatives for the person who doesn't want or can't afford an extended training period.

Therapists and technicians have good to excellent job prospects through the 1980s. The greatest growth will be in the newest areas. Growth will continue in other areas, too, as long as there is not a backlog of trained personnel.

7.

LABORATORY TECHNOLOGIST

It is before seven in the morning, but the heat is already rising heavily from the pavement around the new hospital wing. The pale young maples wave in front of the new brick and tinted glass of the eight-story structure.

Among other things the wing houses a new blood laboratory. A room filled with huge machines is already alive with activity. One hundred laboratory technicians and technologists, mostly young women, set themselves up as the machines roar into action. The blood samples arrive in stainless-steel carts, taken earlier in the morning by phlebotomy teams. The teams are made up of medical students who earn extra money by making the morning blood rounds.

Across the hall from the new blood laboratory, a streamlined elevator slides down to the main floor of the hospital complex. A maze of hallways with brightly colored graphic directions on the walls leads through to the older wings. Here the hospital is four stories high instead of eight. The ceilings are high and the windows narrow and heavily draped. The psychiatric division of the hospital consists of two floors in one of these older wings.

At exactly seven o'clock, Judy Smith opens the door to her second-floor laboratory on the psychiatric wards. She is thirty-four, tall and slender with dark hair pulled back gently from her face. She wears a mint green summer dress and low-heeled shoes. She has a gentle properness that seems almost out of place in this large hospital setting.

"We women like working alone," Judy explains as she sets down her bag and puts her lunch in the small refrigerator. She shares the full-time lab technologist position with another woman, but they work on alternate days. "I've thought of working over there," she gestures in the direction of the new blood laboratory. "I just don't know. That wouldn't be a good situation for me. I like working alone. There has been talk of closing down the satellite labs, like ours, and having everything done at the new lab. Our psychiatric doctors went to bat for us. They want their own lab. They get special service, same day results. At a central lab, they'd have to wait two days or more for a written report, and then it's done by computer and if the cards aren't filled out right, they're lost."

Judy's laboratory is one large room, about thirty by twenty feet. It is a corner room and brighter than most rooms in the old part of the hospital. A marble counter runs through the center of the room, and the walls are lined with counters, wall cabinets, sinks and a variety of machines and racks. It is spotless, and looks very much like a good high-school chemistry laboratory.

"Of course, the equipment in the new wing is pretty fancy. They can take one blood sample, run it through the computer and get about eighteen tests done on it. That's efficient sometimes. But it's also very expensive. We can do blood sugar here and charge the patient five dollars. In the new lab the doctors will routinely run the whole series and charge thirty dollars just because it's there."

Judy puts a white lab coat on over her dress and buttons it carefully. On the center counter a pile of yellow lab request sheets is waiting.

"The tests we do are pretty routine . . . mostly white blood cell counts, blood sugar, urine. There are some other tests we do here, and some samples we take and send to other labs. Our most important test here is the lithium test. There are lots of patients on lithium therapy for manic-depressive psychosis. Some of them have three blood samples drawn a week so their dosages can be regulated. There's great variation among people in how the drug is handled in the body."

She puts the lab orders on a cart stocked with disposable syringes and test tubes and takes the elevator down to the wards. The ward attendant has already gathered most of the patients Judy needs. The patients have been woken for their before-breakfast tests, and they stumble hazily in their bathrobes and pajamas, seating themselves at card tables along the walls. Some look up to greet Judy as she passes them. Many are motionless, eyes distant and vacant. A tall thin man raises his head from a table and smiles at her, drool hanging from the corners of his mouth. He is retarded, Judy explains later, and has tried to commit suicide several times. They don't know what to do with him at home.

"How are you today, Mr. Jackson?" she says to him gently. "Can I get some blood from you this morning?" He rolls up the sleeve of his hospital gown and she wraps some surgical tubing above his elbow. She presses gently around the lower arm. "This is my friend with zero veins," she smiles. Mr. Jackson turns to the other patients and grins proudly. "Let's see." She takes a syringe out of its white paper wrapper and plunges the needle firmly into Mr. Jackson's arm. "Well, there." She loosens the tubing. "We did pretty well this morning. There. You're all done. Andrea, let's see. I've got you today, don't I?"

A young woman seated at the same table looks up. She is an athletically built person with great dark circles under her eyes. She has been in the hospital for almost a month. Her first week she didn't move out of bed.

"You look better today," Judy says as she puts on the tubing.

"I'm in a better mood," Andrea says. "I guess I was pretty nasty yesterday."

"Well, you weren't too friendly." Judy smiles. "I'm glad you're feeling better."

A well-groomed middle-aged man is sitting in a lounge chair in a handsome corduroy bathrobe. He barely acknowledges Judy as she approaches, but rolls up his sleeve and turns his head away.

"How are you feeling, Mr. Whitney?" she asks, but there is no answer. Judy does a half dozen more patients. She moves slowly and speaks slowly and gently to all of them. Her handling of the patients seems not intimate, but humane.

"Mr. Whitney," she explains, moving the cart across the hall to another ward, "is a prominent businessman in another city. This is his third stay in two years. This time, he's been in for two months. Manic-depressive is the diagnosis. He's one of our lithium patients. When I first started working here, we'd see these great recoveries and the nurses would all say 'They'll be back.' It seems like a lot of them do come back."

The other ward is brighter, sunshine filtering through the dusty windows. The group is livelier and they greet Judy robustly as she wheels in her cart.

"Here comes the vampire!" someone calls out.

"Let's get this going. We want to go to breakfast."

"All right. I'll get to you as soon as I can." She parks her cart at a big round table next to a heavy woman in her sixties.

"Emma, how are you this morning?" Emma offers her arm resolutely across the table.

"Not too bad. Gee, yesterday we went bowling. Today I think we go somewhere too. Maybe to a movie. Something. We're going on the bus. Ouch!"

"Oh, I'm awfully sorry. We've been getting so many bad needles in this last batch. Sometimes I think we should go back to the reusable ones. But then, there are conveniences and the disposables are guaranteed sterile. There we go . . . we got it this time." She empties the syringe into the test tube and wraps the lab order around it with a rubber band.

"Mr. Chelsea?" A young man, a teenager, comes up. He is short and blond, his face badly scarred. "This is your lithium blood test, isn't it?" The man nods. "I'll be drawing two more samples from you this week. We need to do that to make sure you are getting the right amount of medication."

"OK," he replies.

Judy heads back to the elevator with her cart. "Mr. Chelsea is another attempted suicide. I get to know some of the patients fairly well. I may miss some patients because of our alternating work schedule, but most of them are here for a while. Sometimes it makes your job harder to know about the patient histories. Last month there was a fellow here who killed his baby son. I was pretty nervous. But he was as calm as you please. You'd never have picked him out as a violent person. We do have problems sometimes in the quiet room. That's where they put patients who are too hard to handle. They have a guard there, Bruce. He's an older fellow. I think he drinks a bit, but he's awfully strong. He's just not always there when you need him. I was taking a sample one day and the patient seemed all right. I thought he was pretty well sedated. All of a sudden he grabbed me by the throat and started choking me. Bruce got there, but not a minute too soon." Judy laughs lightly, as though she were talking about putting too much salt in a recipe. "I was OK, though. It didn't bother me too much."

She opens the door to the lab and wheels in her cart.

"I like to get the lithium tests started first. They take the longest, and I like to finish all the early tests around the same time." She takes a rack of tubes to a dispenser and adds an automatically measured amount of clear liquid to each empty tube. The serum is then measured and added.

"The tests are pretty much cookbook tests. We follow the procedures outlined in the manuals. Every test has a duplicate run with it, plus, to start, we have to run a control to make sure the machines and chemical agents are working correctly." Now she sets a rack of tubes in a centrifuge and turns it on. "You could approach this job in several different ways. Someone who had a real interest in biochemistry could get involved in that aspect of it. They could become the scientists and discoverers of the field. I'm more interested in the patient care. I do just as good a job with the tests, but I may not understand all the chemistry of how it works."

There is a knock on the door and a young doctor comes in with a blood sample and a requisition.

"You can set it on the rack there," Judy says. The doctor sets the tubes in a rack with the others and walks out. Judy lowers her voice a little. "That's what we call a mystery sample... just a number, no name. It could be someone on the staff of the hospital who's on lithium therapy and doesn't want it to get around. We don't know." She begins another series of tests at another station in the lab. "It does bother me a bit. With Mr. Whitney downstairs, for example, the doctors tell him it's nothing to be ashamed of, you don't have to hide it, there's no stigma attached to manic-depressive breakdowns anymore. But then one of them gets sick and they are afraid, even among the people who should understand best."

A buzzer goes off on the centrifuge and she steps back to take the tubes out.

"It can get awfully rushed here. But it is nice to run the lab alone. The other woman who shares this job used to work with me. We got along fine, but in a way it was less efficient. We were always bumping into each other and things wouldn't get done because we'd think the other one was doing it. When we stopped doing research projects and just did clinical lab work, our work load lessened and we decided to split the job. We each feel independent and we have whole days to spend with our families when we need them. We divide the management tasks. Sue is in charge of ordering certain things, and I pick certain things up. It's worked out well. We used to be the only place in the hospital that could do a lithium test. That meant we had to be on call every night and weekends for emergencies. Now they have a backup machine in the new lab and we're relieved of that responsibility."

There is a knock at the door and a nurse comes in with a urine sample. She smiles at Judy.

"How long will it take?"

"Oh, before noon, I hope," Judy says. "Maybe not that early. I'll call you."

"Great. Wish me luck."

"Oh, I do, Eleanor." The nurse leaves. "I told her I'd do a pregnancy test for her this morning. Poor thing has been trying to get pregnant for over a year now. I sympathize with her. It took me a long time to get pregnant with my kids too."

The phone rings. One of the ward clerks is calling. A doctor wants a blood sample taken from a patient for research purposes. The sample must be hemolyzed and dark and cold.

"Can you bring me a thermos or something?" Judy asks. "I don't have anything right here to keep it cold ... Well, all right. I'll think of something." The patient comes and Judy draws the sample quickly and wraps it in several paper towels and then in a plastic bag. She puts the bag in a styrofoam cup with cracked ice around it. "I think I shook it up enough to hemolyze it. That means rupturing the red blood cells."

She goes back to her regular blood tests, but is interrupted again. A tanned, cheerful man comes in for a blood test. He seems to be dressed for the golf course.

"Well, I'm glad we got this straightened out," Judy greets him.

"It's like a game of telephone, you know," the man says. "He said 'Don't take it Monday' and I thought he said 'Don't take it until Monday.'"

"Well, this should take care of it." Judy finishes drawing his sample. "Have a good day now."

"Same to you." The gentleman leaves.

"He's an outpatient on lithium. One of the doctors here sees him. I did a blood test on him Monday and there was no lithium in his sample. So I redid it twice, and still no lithium. When the reports went out, the doctor's secretary called me and said there must be some mistake. I said I didn't think so, but I did two more tests anyway and there was no lithium. I called her back. Well, she got a bit huffy and said the doctor said that it was impossible ... there must be a mistake. I tried once more and then the doctor called and he was huffy. I told him all the other tests were going normally so I didn't think there was a problem in the lab. The patient came in that afternoon and there was a misunderstanding about his drug sequence. He hadn't started to take lithium until after I drew his sample. We have very few problems with the doctors really. They're very cooperative and thankful that we're here. They have so little control when they send things to the new lab."

Judy goes back to her tests again. Outpatients arrive through the morning. At ten o'clock several diabetics come up together for their second sugar of the day. The early morning test is done as a fasting test. The tests at ten and at two are planned to be two hours after meals.

"I feel a little more pressure today than usual. I have to get away early to go to a funeral, and that means getting records written up and filed by three. I'm grateful for the days off in between. I kind of build up steam.

"I've been working for sixteen years now, and I've had several different jobs. My high school had a cooperative education program, and I got to work half-time in a hospital lab. After graduation, I was on a three-year in-service training program at the same hospital. I went to college at nights and almost finished two years of a bachelor's degree in medical technology. Then I quit to get married and moved 400 miles.

"The requirements to be a laboratory technologist now are a bachelor's degree and a one-year internship. You also have to pass boards. The lab technicians usually need two years of training now. There are also lab assistants who get trained in a special area rather than in the broad field.

"My own training was on the job, with some college training, as well. I try to keep up with changes in the field. There are often continuing education courses available, either through the hospitals or other agencies.

"The technologists in the new lab don't have the patient contact and I don't think they have the sense of purpose I have. I think they prefer it that way. They think I'm crazy for putting up with the hassles here . . . all the responsibility, and I don't get paid any more than they do. They have their sick days and personal business days. We haven't taken a sick day all year. It's an inconvenience to my partner, who would have to come in to cover for me. We have to work extra to cover for each other's vacations too. We can't just hang a Closed sign up on the door. Over in the new lab, the techs sit at one machine doing one thing all day and it's easy to get substitutes.

"I think it's too bad the educational requirements are so heavy now. People go through all that schooling and it's hard to turn back if they don't like the work. I'd go for more on-the-job training and less classroom work. All the new certification business, though, has come directly out of the Medicare scandals in private labs a few years back."

When the blood sugar tests are done and recorded, Judy checks back to the pregnancy test she started and shakes her head. "Can't see anything yet. I thought I might try to call Eleanor before she left for lunch." Judy takes her own lunch out of the icebox and makes herself some tea on a Bunsen burner.

"I went back to work quite soon after my children were born. They're fourteen and twelve now. I love my family life and I wasn't forced back to work because of money. But I really missed it. After my first baby was born, I started working part-time with four internists, running their office laboratory. By the time my second baby came I was working ten hours a day. It was a very interesting job, but the pace was exhausting. So much pressure, and very few benefits. When I changed to a hospital job one of the internists said, 'You'll be back. You won't be able to sit on a lab stool all day like they do.' But it wasn't like that. I worked in the newborn intensive-care nursery, taking oxygen blood levels on babies with heart problems. I did that for three years. It was emotionally draining, but exciting. I assisted in heart catheterizations with the infants, and did the blood gases. In tight situations I had to do all kinds of things. One time they were using a defibrillator on a baby. I reached over the stainless-steel table to help and one of the doctors practically knocked me across the room. I guess I could have been badly shocked if I'd touched the table. Well . . ." she shrugs her shoulders with a smile and stirs into her tea. The phone rings on her desk. It is the ward clerk from the first ward. She wants to know what patients are due for a third blood sugar. Judy checks her charts and reads off the names.

"The ward clerks make such a big difference. They aren't paid very well and the turnover is high. When you get a new one it's tough. Patients are gone when you need them, records get misplaced. Everything is wild. A good ward clerk makes the job easy for us. Teamwork is really important."

An older woman in a white pants suit comes back to Judy's desk. She is the hospital beautician.

"Mrs. Barnes helps the women keep themselves up and gives the men haircuts too," Judy says. "It helps morale."

"What can you tell me about mono?" Mrs. Barnes asks. "I think my son has it."

"Well, I can look it up for you." Judy gets up and goes to the bookshelves at one corner of the lab. "But you ought to get him to a doctor. A blood test is the only way to tell for sure."

"I can't get him to a doctor. He's been worn out for weeks and complaining and his wife can't get him to go and I can't either."

Judy reads the definition of mononucleosis out of the medical dictionary. "Maybe you could get him to come in. I could get a sample taken but he'd still have to see a doctor."

"Well, I'll work on him. Maybe I can get him to come in here. I might draw the blood myself with my teeth, he's so stubborn."

"Have a nice day, Mrs. Barnes."

"You too, Judy."

Judy finishes lunch between outpatient visits. Then she goes on to the last stage of the lithium test, which is done in the flame photometer. With a pipette, she suctions blood out of the test tubes and mixes it with another liquid in little paper cups. The cups are placed in the photometer and the results read off a gauge and recorded. Two samples are done on each patient.

"Most lab workers have at least one bad experience with a pipette. That should be all it takes to learn not to get it in your mouth. You'd think urine would be the most dangerous, but it usually isn't. I got spinal fluid in my mouth, on my first job. If the patient had had meningitis or encephalitis, I would have been in trouble. But, luckily he didn't."

Judy makes a note to order more pipettes on a sheet kept on the counter.

"We used to have a salesman come here to the lab on a regular basis. They'd get whatever we wanted in two days, just with a phone call. Now they have a new purchasing system. Everything has to go through one office. It takes ages to get anything."

Judy finishes up the other tests and gets them recorded on her own list. Two more outpatients come and she draws samples and gets the tests started. In between steps she takes time to call Eleanor about the pregnancy test.

"It looks negative, Eleanor. Of course, it's still early. You might bring another sample next week . . . OK, I'm sorry."

"I spent quite a bit of time in hospitals when I was a kid," Judy says. "I have first-hand experience with what pleasant personnel can do. As for myself I try to be gentle and accurate, to keep in mind what the work is for."

Judy's day is almost over. Her final concern is to record the lab results in the charts downstairs. Gathering up her things, she heads for the office. Taking out each chart, she carefully writes the information and then replaces the chart in the files. Once finished, she takes off her lab coat and adjusts the collar of her dress. Picking up her pocketbook, she pauses briefly in front of the office mirror. She looks the same as she did when she came to work . . . fresh, clean, orderly.

"Mental illness is still such a stigma. I don't know a whole lot about it. But there is evidence now that it may be a result of chemical imbalance. Just chemicals. All that suffering in a lifetime. Looking at it that way, I know I'm not immune. It could be me."

SUMMARY

DUTIES: *The lab technologist performs relatively complex chemical, microscopic and bacteriological diagnostic tests. In the small laboratory, the technologist may perform a wide range of tests, while in a large laboratory s/he is apt to specialize.* Lab technicians *may perform many of the same tests as the technologist, but without the same depth of knowledge and correspondingly less independence.* Lab assistants *work under a technician or technologist, usually concentrating on one area or routine.*

TRAINING: *The lab technologist requires four years of training in a regular BS liberal-arts program. The technicians usually have two years of training from a community college or technical school, while a certified lab assistant requires only one year of training. For more information, contact:*

> *American Society for Medical Technology*
> *5555 West Loop South*
> *Bellaire, Texas 77401*

SALARY: *$10,500 to start. Lab assistants start at $7,600. The technicians' salaries range between the two.*

8

OPERATING ROOM TECHNICIAN

It is just before seven at a large university teaching hospital. In a locker room across the hall from the second-floor operating suite, Marie Morgan sheds her street clothes for green hospital garb, and covers her shoes with special paper booties.

Marie has just come back from a week's vacation and her skin is bronze. She has bright blue eyes with heavy dark lashes, and black hair. Even with the green hood over her hair, her coloring is striking. Other nurses and technicians dress too, each putting on an identifying hood—white for the registered nurses, green for the operating room technicians, blue for students.

Locking away her street clothes for the day, Marie crosses the hall through the swinging door marked Operating Room Personnel Only. Inside is a broad hallway, with rooms to each side. An elderly patient on a cart in the hall lies quietly, gazing at the white ceiling. Smells of coffee drift from the lounge.

"We share the lounge with the doctors," Marie whispers. "It's kind of nice. This way we're able to question them about procedures. Some of the other operating areas don't do that."

Marie is going into her fourth year of work as an operating room technician in this hospital. She has worked almost the whole time in otolaryngology, the area concerned with the ear, nose and throat.

"When I first came, I had to go through all the different services —gynecology, general surgery, orthopedics—so I can fill in when they need me. We have to work weekends every five weeks. That's all emergency surgery, so you have to know what all of the setups are. I'm also on call at least once a week.

"Here," she points to a printed notice on the wall of the lounge.

"We get the schedule of surgery a day in advance. I'm in operating room two. We usually have one nurse and one OR Tech (operating room technician) in each room. We'll have an extra nurse today because there's a student. Lynn?" she turns to a woman in a white nurse's hood. "Are the patients late today, or what?"

"I think I hear our first one now. The tonsils and adenoids. Are you scrubbing?"

"If it's OK with you." Marie goes into the scrub room. She grabs a mask from a box and puts it on quickly. Then she takes a plastic wrapped sponge, basted in surgical soap, from a shelf. "You always have to have one person scrubbing and one person circulating. The circulating person can go in and out to get supplies, medications, do paper work, but can't touch anything that is sterile. The person who scrubs stays sterile and does all the instrument passing."

Marie begins scrubbing, working from the fingers up to above her elbows. A special stick in the kit is used under the fingernails.

"We are supposed to do five rounds of scrubbing at the beginning of each day. That means five complete scrubs on each arm. Between operations we do three. If we've been on vacation for any length of time, we're supposed to do ten to start with." She goes around a corner and through the swinging doors into the operating room. She dries her hands with a green sterile cloth, then puts on an operating gown with long sleeves. Lynn helps her into the gown and then opens a package of gloves for her, without touching the gloves themselves.

"When you work in the same place for a while, the routine gets automatic. Still, you get mixed up sometimes, switching between scrubbing and circulating. If you make a mistake it sometimes means stripping down and starting a setup all over again."

Marie briskly sets up her table for the adenoid and tonsil operation. Most of the instruments she needs are already in sterile packages. She spreads sterile sheets over the tables, then carefully lines up the various instruments, clamps, scissors, knives and sponges. She screws special sterile handles onto the overhead lamps so the surgeon can adjust the light.

"We set the tables up pretty much according to a written list of what is needed for a standard operation. Sometimes you may know a particular doctor uses other instruments, and you make sure she or he has them. Each tech may set up a bit differently. On this operation we'll be working with a resident. Dr. Carbon is from New Zealand and I sometimes can't understand what he says."

Dr. Carbon brushes through the door. His arms, bent at the elbows, are dripping with water. He is a large man with blondish hair and freckles.

"God has arrived," he says with a heavy accent. "Let there be some bloody light." Lynn turns on one of the overhead lights. Marie hands him a sterile towel, then gets a gown. Lynn ties up the back of the gown without contaminating it. "Is the patient here yet?"

"No. I hear him out there though," Marie says. "Lynn, you go. They're trying to get him away from his mother. That's the hardest part." Lynn goes out and comes back in. An orderly is pushing the cart. A blond, three-year-old boy is sitting up on the cart screaming. Lynn stands by trying to comfort him.

"Wanna go home!" he wails. "I want my mom!"

The anesthesiologist, a middle-aged woman, is training a medical student today. There is a great deal of noise, between the child crying, Lynn comforting and the anesthesiologist trying to explain things to both her student and the child.

"That's one thing about a teaching hospital," Marie says. "Everything takes a little longer. There are always students in on things. The cases are sometimes more interesting, though, because you get a lot of cases that local doctors won't handle."

The child is put to sleep inhaling the anesthetic gases through a mask. The anesthesiologist is trying to teach the student to insert the endotracheal tube which the child will breathe through during the operation. The student is having problems. Dr. Carbon taps his toes and looks at the clock.

"I'm sorry, sir," the student looks up nervously.

"Let's get on with it," he says.

"Just a few more minutes," the anesthesiologist asks. The student makes a final attempt and succeeds.

The doctor moves his chair over to the patient's head. Lynn pushes Marie's table and a sterile draped stool next to it. Lynn puts a stocking cap on the child's hair. Marie passes sterile towels to the doctor to go around the cap. The eyes are taped to avoid possible injury.

As the operation begins, Marie hands the doctor sterile packing, mirrors, the suction hose to remove blood from the throat and various cutting instruments. She leans over the table to watch more closely.

"Doing a good job means anticipating," Marie says. "That's what they keep telling you in school. When you go through the same operation several times, you get good at it."

The adenoids come out first, little pieces of tissue. Then the tonsils, larger pieces. Marie picks them up in her gloved hand and drops them into the lab cup Lynn holds out.

"These are examined by pathologists routinely," Marie explains. "It's a legal requirement, just in case."

"There, that takes care of the bleeding," Dr. Carbon says, drawing out the long gauze packing. "Some patients go back to their rooms with some oozing. Makes me nervous. I like it all to stop here." The medical student removes the tube. The doctor removes the drapes and tosses them to Marie who puts them in the laundry hamper. The child leaves the room while Marie and Lynn strip the tables for the next operation.

"An atticotomy and placement of drain tubes is the next operation," Marie says. "This is done with a microscope. It'll be a fairly long operation. If they're doing an operation I haven't done before, I'll read up on it the night before. With these microscopic ear surgeries, I know basically what the procedures are, but looking into the microscope I can't understand much. They'll have a fifth-year resident in on this," she adds. "Dr. Carbon is first year. They don't let the first year residents do major ear surgery."

When the room is stripped down, Marie dumps her gown, mask and gloves and goes to the lounge for coffee. The surgical personnel are not allowed to leave the floor during the day, so coffee and sweet rolls are provided in the lounge. The lounge is a narrow room crowded with doctors, nurses and technicians. There is a sudden silence when a short pudgy man of about fifty enters. He is slightly balding. When he speaks, it is with a heavy German accent.

"And who will work with me today?" He smiles, taking a roll offered by a nurse. Two hands go up. "Anna and Paula . . . good. We will do something special today." He beams at his helpers.

"That's Dr. Hoffritz," Marie whispers when he leaves. "He's a plastic surgeon, world famous. He's sort of the plum of the surgical staff. Difficult to work with sometimes. Most of the doctors are nice, but you do get some who like to chew out the nursing staff. Most of them only do it when they're in a tight spot, when things aren't going well. They can lash out, but if they're in the wrong, they may apologize later. In a teaching hospital, with so many people at different levels of training, I feel pretty comfortable speaking out. I've been here a while, and I'm supposed to be an expert on sterile procedures. I feel all right pointing things out now and then. If a doctor touches the bottom of his chair, or scratches his head, I'll offer him a new glove. One time a resident was about to inject a local anesthetic and the concentration he was using was too much. I said, 'Dr. Adams doesn't use that much.' He argued with me but I was stubborn. I said, 'Look, I know he doesn't use that much.' So he finally broke down and checked. I was right. You just have to know when to say something and when to keep quiet, common sense.

"I went into the OR tech program because a friend of mine told me about it. There was one at a community college near my home. It's only a year. I just couldn't afford more than that, or I might have gone into nursing. Actually I only did nine months. The university hospital called my teacher and asked if there were any techs ready for hiring, so she let me go early.

"We had about three months of classroom training and book learning ... anatomy, principles of sterile techniques and sterile procedures. The rest of the time was spent working at local hospitals in the operating rooms, with classes one day a week."

Marie finishes her roll and goes back to scrub for the next operation.

"I had never had any experience with sick people until I scrubbed my first case. My mother said, 'Oh it will be awful, you're so squeamish.' But there was nothing to it. I was so nervous about doing my job, so intent on doing the right thing, that I just didn't have time to think about anything else. You don't get to know the patients personally, like you would on the wards, but still you must treat each one as if he were a member of your own family. That way you're always doing your best."

Another mother-child separation is going on in the hall as Marie brushes through the swinging doors with wet hands. Lynn brings in another three-year-old boy. The anesthesiologist and her student work quickly with the child. The student puts the tube down effortlessly. Marie sets her table up quickly. It is a bigger table with more instruments.

"When they are working with the microscope, you have to place the instruments in their hands the way they'll use them so they don't have to take their eyes off the scope. The less movement in passing instruments, the better." The microscope itself is draped in special cloths to allow the surgeon to handle the adjustments.

Dr. Carbon comes in scrubbed with Dr. Wyatt, a fifth-year resident, behind him. Lynn and Marie get them gowned and gloved. The ear and surrounding skin surface of the little boy are scrubbed with surgical soap and dried. The eyelids are taped shut and Marie drapes sterile towels and sheets around the ear, creating a sterile field.

Dr. Wyatt takes a clear plastic drape, like a large piece of Scotch tape, and presses it around the exposed face and ear. He then seats himself next to the child's head; Dr. Carbon is slightly above it. The microscope has a special side arm to allow for an observer.

Dr. Wyatt selects the right size speculum, a small metal funnel that fits in the ear. The view inside the ear is like a glistening wet anatomical drawing. The operation is delicate and there is little room for error in the small picture the microscope shows. Dr. Wyatt works steadily for an hour, with only an occasional soft question from Dr. Carbon. Marie leans over the table to within a few inches of Dr. Wyatt's hand to take and pass instruments.

Another doctor breezes into the room. He is in his late thirties and has a youthful, athletic bounce to his walk. He is wearing less-than-white gym shoes with his green surgical suit.

"Hi, Dr. Adams," Marie whispers through her mask. Her eyebrows raise a bit at the shoes, but she doesn't say anything. Dr. Carbon backs away from his viewing position and Dr. Adams looks in.

"You're doing well," Dr. Adams says, his voice low and steady. "You're going to have to move back a bit more on it . . . that's it. Now see . . ." He pulls a pen from his shirt pocket and draws a quick sketch on his pants. "That's what you want. Don't rush it. You're doing fine. Let's watch that nerve ending there . . . That's it. I'll be right outside if you need me."

Dr. Adams leaves, and Dr. Wyatt goes on with his work. "Keep an eye on the cheek please, Lynn," he says. "Tell me if you see any twitching from that nerve."

"We have operations that go on for twelve hours sometimes," Marie says. "You could just die trying to concentrate. There'll be a pause where there is nothing for you to do. Then all of a sudden you'll hear a doctor asking for something and you realize you're a hundred miles away." After another half an hour, Dr. Adams comes back in, scrubbed. Lynn helps him into a gown and gloves. Dr. Wyatt moves over to the viewing position and Dr. Adams finishes up a stage of the surgery.

"There. You can go in and get the fascia now," Dr. Adams says, and leaves again.

"I'll need the local," Dr. Wyatt says. Marie passes the filled syringe. He injects it behind the exposed ear. He makes an incision, with Marie handing instruments in a steady stream. He removes a piece of the tough, plastic-like membrane next to the muscle. This will be used to strengthen the ear drum. The piece is about a half an inch square. He passes it to Marie who takes it in her gloved hand. "The blood looks a little dark," Dr. Wyatt says to the anesthesiologist. "Is the patient getting enough oxygen?" She nods.

Marie cleans off the piece of fascia and flattens it on two tongue depressors. She puts it in a metal clamp and squeezes it, then sets it to dry in front of a lamp. Dr. Wyatt is asking for suture materials to close the incision.

"That was nice of you not to yell at Helen the other day," Marie says to Dr. Wyatt.

"I guess. How the hell do you lose a piece of fascia?"

"She'd never scrubbed for one of those cases before. She almost died. God, it must have been awful," Marie laughs. Dr. Wyatt shakes his head.

"Lynn, I need a new glove," Marie says. She has poked a hole in one of her gloves with a needle. Lynn is there quickly, holding out the opened package of gloves and taking the contaminated needle. With the glove changed, Marie takes a paper punch from her tray and punches out a dozen circles from a piece of white material used for packing the ear canal.

"This is gelfoam," she explains. "It expands in the body moisture and then dissolves slowly. They use it to hold the fascia in place."

The fascia is put through the funnel into the ear. Marie passes the dots of gelfoam with special long tweezers.

"Do you have the tubes ready, Marie? I'll need them in a minute."

"Right."

"I'll be closing in five minutes," Dr. Wyatt tells the anesthesiologist. Marie passes him the little plastic tubes that go through the ear drum.

"Sometimes we'll spend a whole day just doing tube operations. Lots of little kids get them now if they have chronic ear infections. It helps with drainage."

"Bobby," the anesthesiologist calls. "Wake up, Bobby." The child is wheeled out of the room as the doctors take off their gowns.

"We can eat lunch now," Marie says. "We can have it sent up from the cafeteria. Actually, I hardly ever eat anything until evening. Bad habit." Marie settles into a chair in the lounge. She gets a cup of coffee and lights a cigarette. Dr. Wyatt steps into the lounge with a sandwich in one hand.

"That's a nice habit too," he says, pointing to the cigarette. "But never mind. When you need surgery, just make sure you come to me. I'll do good work." Marie waves an impatient hand at him.

"We do all the throat cases here," Marie explains. "Throat cancer, removing larynges . . . those can be long operations. We usually only see a patient once while he's here for surgery. Some are sent from other parts of the state with a special problem. We do get to know some, though . . . patients who become a kind of triumph. We had a guy a few years ago who fell out of his motor boat and had his face run over by the propeller. He's had numerous operations here. Gradually we reconstructed his ear, then a little of his cheek, then his chin. When Dr. Hoffritz gets finished with all the surgeries, the patient will look like a new man. Or the cleft lip and palate children. They are usually here for several operations. That's real miracle surgery too. It's rewarding."

"Are you ready to scrub?" Lynn calls from the doorway.

"I was thinking about it." Marie starts to get up.

"I don't know if they're going to do this case or not. He's got a bad cough. They may cancel."

Marie peeks into the operating room on her way to scrub. Two nurses are trying to move a man from the cart to the operating table. He is in his sixties, with a great bulging stomach, his face blotchy.

"Oh my God!" he yells from the fog of his sedation. "Oh God!" Marie moves quickly to give the nurses a hand.

"All right, Bart," Marie says. "We're going to roll you a bit. Try not to thrash around so much."

"Oh no!" Bart yells.

They finally get him onto the operating table. The anesthesiologist rushes to his side. His arm is covered with blood.

"He's pulled out his IV," she says quietly. A nurse quickly undoes the tape and cleans the arm.

"It's OK, Bart. They're going to put it back in. Just a minute now." The anesthesiologist puts the needle in quickly, with two nurses holding Bart's arm. Marie stands on the opposite side, holding his other hand in hers.

When Bart is finally calm, Marie leaves to scrub. Dr. Wyatt, Dr. Carbon and a third resident, Dr. Hand, are checking the patient's vital signs.

"Are you going to go ahead?" Marie asks as she comes back in.

"Yes. Things seem pretty stable now," Dr. Carbon says.

Marie's table is very large for this operation.

"This is a partial neck," she explains. "They are going to look at an enlarged lymph node. They'll have it biopsied. If it's cancerous, lymphoma, they'll close up. They have to run all kinds of tests to see the extent of the disease. If it isn't lymphoma, they'll go ahead with a longer exploratory operation. We set up for the longer one in advance."

The patient is sedated and draped. Dr. Carbon takes a marking pen from Marie to map out the incision they will make.

"That line should be shorter," Dr. Hand says to Dr. Carbon. "It should be a gentle curve, around this way." He points.

"That *is* a gentle curve," Dr. Carbon says.

"It doesn't look like a gentle curve to me."

Marie laughs. The three doctors are standing at the neck. Marie's large table is over Bart's chest, and she stands on a high step stool on the side, leaning over to pass instruments.

"Count these with me," Marie says to Lynn quietly. Marie counts out the sponges on the table and Lynn nods. "We have to count all the sponges and cotton balls in advance to make sure everything is accounted for at the end of the case. The OR techs are allowed to count cotton balls themselves, but we have to have a nurse to count the sponges with us. In some hospitals even the instruments must be counted."

The doctors have exposed the swollen lymph node and are trying to ease it out.

"Damn. I should be doing this more quickly. I can't seem to . . ."

"Take it easy. I've found if you work around to the back . . . There . . . it's coming now."

"There it comes," Dr. Wyatt pulls out the node, a yellowish, round piece of tissue about the diameter of a quarter. "Is the pathologist here?"

"I called him ten minutes ago," Lynn says.

Lynn holds out a container for the specimen and puts a lid on it with the patient's name. The man from the lab arrives to take it from her.

"I'm going to go ahead and close," Dr. Wyatt says. "It may be twenty minutes before we get the word. If it's lymphoma we'll be all done. If it isn't, we'll just snip the stitches."

Marie begins handing the suture materials to Dr. Wyatt. The incision, about eight inches down the side of the neck, is gradually closed. Then the phone rings. They all turn expectantly as Lynn answers the phone.

"It's lymphoma," she says as she hangs up.

"Now he'll go through staging," Marie explains as Dr. Wyatt puts in the final stitches. "That means a series of tests to pinpoint the extent of the disease. Lymphoma can respond well to chemical therapy if it's not too far along."

Marie strips down the operating room for the day.

"Occasionally we'll have a cancellation or short cases. Then we'll have time to work cleaning instruments. If things are really slow we might get sent to one of the other operating rooms, but that doesn't happen often. The hospital has a job description printed for technicians. The OR techs have listed as their primary responsibility "Transporting Patients." But we usually only help get patients for first cases in the morning.

"I still think sometimes of going into nurse's training. But I like working here and I'm not that anxious to change. It would be good for me financially though. The nurses make twice as much as we do. In the operating room, the only things they do that we can't are administer medications, take blood pressures and chart records. It's easy to see why a big hospital would want to use OR techs instead of nurses, budgets being what they are.

"My supervisor really likes RNs. If she got the funds, she'd probably like to have all RNs here. When she wrote up my work evaluation last month, she asked if I ever considered going into nursing. I'd do it if I could, but there's no way I can stop working now to do that.

"But that's OK. I feel I'm good at what I do here. In many private hospitals, nurses only circulate while the techs scrub, but being scrubbed in and passing instruments is what I enjoy most."

SUMMARY

DUTIES: *Also known as the surgical technician. The operating room technician assists the surgical team. The OR tech passes instruments during surgery, assists in clean-up and transfer of patients and helps maintain sterile procedures in the operating room.*

TRAINING: *Some OR techs are trained on the job, but a vocational-technical school course is recommended. A high-school diploma is usually required for admission to a program. For more information, contact:*

> *American Society of Allied Health Professionals*
> *1 DuPont Circle NW, Suite 300*
> *Washington, D.C. 20036*

SALARY: *$7,400 is the average starting salary.*

9

RESPIRATORY THERAPIST

It is nine o'clock in the morning. Jean Tanner wheels a machine into a third-floor room of the small Catholic hospital where she works. She passes the first bed. An elderly woman sitting in a chair looks up expectantly. She wheels the machine over to the second bed and plugs a hose into the oxygen supply.

A large old woman lies on the bed. She has a sheet half draped over her torso, but her feet are bare, calloused and discolored. She is asleep, her head thrown back. She breathes heavily. She has white hair, but it is so thin her scalp shows through everywhere. Jean takes off her white lab jacket and puts it at the end of the bed. She leans over the woman's face.

"Emma, good morning!" Jean shouts. "I'm here to give you your breathing exercises." She puts her hands on either side of Emma's face. Emma's eyes half open, then close. "Emma, hon. I'm going to do your breathing exercises now. Let's see if you can give me some nice big breaths, hon." Still no response.

"Emma is eighty, I think," Jean explains. "She had a stroke about a week ago. She hasn't really regained consciousness yet, but she is showing a little alertness now. Seems to understand a bit. The doctor added IPPB therapy four times a day. That's what this machine does: Intermittent Positive Pressure Breathing. It forces humidified oxygen into the lungs. With a stroke patient, getting no activity, you have rapid degeneration of the lung capacity, collapsed sacs and things like that. She already has some mild damage."

The woman in the next bed has rung her nurse's bell.

"Yes?" a nurse comes in on the intercom.

The woman mumbles a reply.

"What?" says the nurse.

"I need a bowel movement," the woman says loudly.

"All right. Someone will be right down."

Jean takes a black face mask from a bag that hangs on the IPPB machine and connects it to the machine's hoses. A nurse comes in and closes the curtain around the neighboring lady's bed.

"All right now, Emma. You remember how this goes. Let's try a deep breath!" Jean glances at her watch. "We usually do about fifteen minutes of treatment. But we have to be careful about signs of fatigue. There are doctors who believe the therapy is a mistake ... that it is just too traumatic having air forced in like that." She places the mask tightly over Emma's mouth with both hands and waits for the old woman to inhale.

"Good. Another deep one now. Good."

After nine minutes Jean stops and takes a stethoscope out of her lab coat pocket. She listens to Emma's heart and takes a pulse. An elderly man walks in and quietly seats himself at the end of the bed.

"Good morning," Jean says.

"Good morning," the man says. A nurse has entered and is checking the three intravenous bottles that are strung above Emma's bed. "How is she today?" he asks the nurse. "About the same?"

"Oh well, I guess so. She is a bit more alert. She's been awake a bit more."

"OK Emma, we're going to do a little more deep breathing now. Just a few more minutes and then we'll finish up." Jean puts the black rubber mask in place again. "This is the most tiring part. With a patient who's alert you can give them a mouthpiece. But with a stroke patient you have to use the mask and push to make sure you have a good seal." Jean finishes and takes a pulse and heart rate again. "Good now, Emma. We'll be back later for some more, hon."

As Jean disconnects the oxygen hose the old man walks to the bedside and leans over.

"Hello, dear," he says softly. "How are you today?"

Jean takes the IPPB machine back to the cardiopulmonary office. One of the other therapists, Barb Michaels, is trying to put together another IPPB machine.

"Do you know where the adapters are for this?" Barb asks as Jean walks in.

"They should be here. No, they're all gone. I'll call Supply. I need some cups for the vaporizer too."

RESPIRATORY THERAPIST

"While you're at it, call Dr. Hickley. See what he wants done for this patient. I can't read the order."

Jean is on the phone for a few minutes. She is acting today as an informal work organizer. There are a total of eleven respiratory therapists, working different shifts, but a third of them work part-time and are usually students who need training assistance. She goes to a back lab room and washes a face mask for Barb to use.

"You're going to Oscar?" she asks.

"Yes. I'll take Sandy with me. She's never done this before. Then I've got a treadmill test here." Barb leaves the office.

"Barb gets kind of a raw deal in a way," Jean explains as she writes up her third set of records on Emma's treatment. "She is classified as a secretary here. She does a lot of the paper work. But she does the therapy too . . . picked it up on the job. She and I are the only ones who do the treadmill test now. But she still gets paid secretarial wages. It's a bummer. But in a small hospital like this, they just use you where they need you. I started out as a nurse's aide here five years ago. Then I got moved to do EKG, electrocardiograms. Then they combined the EKG department and the pulmonary department so I had to learn to do the respiratory aspect. I guess that's the advantage of working in a hospital like this as opposed to a big one. You have a chance to move around a bit. An energetic person is apt to be used to her or his capacities. I learned to do the treadmill test. They needed it. It's a stress test, and it's used mostly with people who are having heart problems that don't always show up on a routine EKG. I already knew the EKG part. The treadmill part I learned from a manual.

"We'll go over to intensive care and get Mary started on her blow bottles." Jean walks briskly along the hall and through swinging doors that say Positively No Admittance. "The blow bottles are a pretty routine exercise for people after surgery. I call it respiratory hygiene. It exercises the lungs, and helps keep fluid from building up and causing infections."

There are twelve rooms in intensive care which are circled around the nursing station. In front of the nursing station TV monitors, showing each patient's vital signs, flicker continuously. Mary is sitting in a chair by the window with half a dozen tubes and wires strung from her to various bottles and plugs by her bed. She had surgery for ulcers several days before. Three months before that she had a breast removed and six months before that surgery for cancer of the colon. She is eighty-three. She is wearing a flowered bathrobe and her grey hair is immaculately groomed.

"Hello there Mary, how are you today?" Jean smiles.

"Oh well, not so good. This is the worst day I've had. Really. I just don't know what's wrong."

"I'm sorry to hear that. Can I get you to do the blow bottle?"

"Oh I've done them this morning already. And I did them last night too. I think I overdid it. I've got pain in my chest now and I just feel awful."

"Well, we'll just skip it for now. I'll come back and catch you later then."

Jean goes to the nursing station, pulls out Mary's chart and writes that the first treatment of the day was done by the patient.

"Jean Tanner. Jean Tanner. 302." Jean picks up the hospital telephone and dials.

"Why do you need that?" she says. "It's not . . . OK . . . I'll be down in a minute." She picks up her own charts and heads back toward the office. "They want one of the respirators in the surgery recovery room, and they can't get it going."

Back by the cardiopulmonary office one of the part-time therapists is fussing with a machine in the hall.

"Why don't you use the one that's already set up?"

"They say they need this one because of the patient's condition. But I can't find a connector for it."

"I'll see if I can get one from the storage room." Jean pulls two large adjustable wrenches from a drawer and goes into the small storage room. With great effort, she takes a metal connector from another machine and takes it back to the one in the hall. "Ah good, it fits." The phone rings in the office.

"They want the respirator," the student says.

"Tell them I'll be right there." Jean wheels the machine down the hall and through the double doors into the recovery room. It is a large room, empty except for a group of people huddled around a patient at one end. It is an old man. He periodically thrashes on the stretcher and a nurse restrains him at his head.

"It's all right, Ralph," the nurse says. "The surgery is over. Try to relax. It's all right."

"I don't think we'll need it after all," the anesthesiologist says to Jean. "He seems to be doing all right now."

"OK." Jean wheels the machine back down the hall.

"They didn't use it?" the student asks. Jean shakes her head. "Why didn't they start bagging him anyway, instead of rushing for this machine? Aren't you supposed to get them used to the bag before you start on the machine?"

"Well, usually." Jean says. She fills out two of the charge slips for the patients she has seen so far that morning.

"I figure our work is about 50 percent paperwork," she explains. "For every contact we have with a patient, we have to write something at the nursing station, something for the hospital, and something for our own records and then a charge slip too. It seems crazy."

Back on the third floor Jean enters another room. A woman in her early fifties is in traction on the bed. She had a pin put in her leg for injuries after an automobile accident. She has already been in traction for a week. Her blow bottles are on the table next to her, two quart jugs with hoses connecting them from the top.

"Hi Rose, how are things going?"

"Oh not too bad I guess."

"Any word yet on how long they're going to keep you like this?"

"No," Rose says irritably. "The doctor who has been seeing me is waiting for Dr. Langlin to make a decision. Dr. Langlin left for a two-week vacation the day after the surgery. So here I am."

"Oh dear. Isn't that a nuisance. Can you do your bottles for me now?"

"Oh well, I guess so. I'm expecting my husband and my brother and his wife any minute."

"It only takes a couple of minutes. Do it fast and then I'll be out of your way."

"All right. Don't set them on the bed though. I don't want to get it messed up." The patient blows the blue liquid in one bottle into the other, and then changes tubes and blows the water back again. Rose strains to finish, keeping one eye toward the door.

"Thataway, Rose. Have a nice visit with your family now. I'll be back later." Jean puts caps over the mouth pieces to keep them clean, wraps the tubes around the top of the bottle, and goes down to the nursing station to get Rose's records.

"The doctors are terribly spoiled in this hospital. I mean, they are treated like gods. When they show up to make rounds in the morning, the nursing station has all their patients' records in neat piles in their own special part of the counter. If there isn't a nurse standing by to go along with them, if anything is out of order or if they have to wait for anything, it gets kind of hairy. In a large hospital I think this isn't quite as true. The doctors in a large hospital seem a little more aware that they are dependent on other people. They might ask a respiratory therapist, or a nurse, for an opinion now and then. Here we don't talk to the doctors. We just get the therapy orders."

Back at the office Barb is chuckling over a report in front of her.

"You missed a good treadmill test. She started complaining about her breath the minute she stepped on, but her heart rate barely changed at all. I don't know. She didn't get much of a test at all. Then she ran out of here because she had to go shopping." Jean looks quickly at the test results.

"Really, it isn't even a valid test." Jean picks up her clip board to write.

At her coffee break in the hospital cafeteria, Jean eats the breakfast she missed that morning.

"Respiratory therapy is still a new enough area that there are a lot of ways to get into it. A big hospital might require a program from a two-year college. There are quite a few of those. But it's still possible in a smaller place, or a place where they're shorthanded, to learn on the job. They've met recently to decide on certification procedures. I could get my certification now, I think, with the experience I've had. There are some six-week crash courses for people with experience too. Then after you get your certification, you take another test later for your registry. That's the highest certification you can get.

"I guess I got into all this pretty haphazardly. I went to college for a year. What I really wanted to learn was occupational therapy. So I signed up with the Air Force to get into their occupational therapy program. I don't want to be negative or anything. I mean, a lot of people ask me about the military training programs and I try not to be discouraging, but really, your chances of getting into the program you want are not very good. It's all done by computer. The training bases get a print-out of what personnel they need in what areas and that's where you go.

"They put me in Air Traffic Control. I wasn't very happy about it. During boot camp we got some really powerful injections for a whole bunch of things combined. I passed out and had a convulsion right after one of the shots. The Air Force said I had epilepsy and accused me of falsifying my enlistment information. They tried to get me court martialed. I just kind of hung in there. I knew I didn't have epilepsy. My mother had been a patient at Mayo Clinic for a long time and I knew doctors there.

"Eventually I was able to win my battle. Four months had gone by, and when I was back in circulation they didn't want Air Traffic Controllers any more. They wanted Medics. It wasn't occupational therapy, but it was closer. That's where I learned how to do electrocardiograms. So then, after I was married, my husband started school here in town. I took a job as a nurse's aide. When they needed someone to do the EKGs they used me. Then the pulmonary and EKG combined offices so here I am.

"The hierarchy in a hospital like this is amazing. It's almost like a caste system. It really interferes with patient care, I think. For example..." Barb arrives with a cup of coffee and sits down. "Barb did you read the report on that carbon monoxide emergency last week? One of the factories on the other side of town had an air-circulating machine, and it was circulating the air the wrong way and they had all these workers getting poisoned. We heard first that we were going to get five of them here, so we had everything set up. They brought in the first five and then they said there were ten more coming, so we really had to hustle around. It would have been fine... things were going smoothly. But we don't get that many emergencies here. I mean, the heavy trauma cases are usually sent over to the big hospital, so all these people were down here trying to get in on the action—administrators, the head of personnel; they were lined up along the walls pretending they had something to do with it. Then in the write-up they said 'Therapists from cardiopulmonary assisted.' That's annoying."

Jean heads back up to the third floor to do Emma again on the IPPB machine. This time the old woman does not even lift her eyes when Jean speaks to her. She only give a whistling moan as her lungs exhale. Her husband has covered her feet with a light blanket.

"One kind of therapy that is very effective is postural drainage. I don't have any patients on it now," Jean says. "It's more apt to be used during the winter when there are a lot of respiratory infections. It involves tilting the patient downward and palpating sections of the lung that are filled with fluid. I had a fellow in here last winter with pneumonia in his right lung. I spent some time on postural drainage in the lower sections of that side and God, he coughed up about a cup of green gunk. It's also something you can teach the patient to do at home on his own." Jean stops to check Emma's breathing before going on with the treatment. "We have a heavy dose of elderly people here. As far as really gory situations, we just don't see them. They are usually sent to the larger hospitals. We get lots of old people. But I can tell just since I've worked here, there is an increase in respiratory cases, people who can be assisted by our therapies. It's terrible to look forward to, but I'm sure it's going to be a continuing trend, with all the air pollution. Our lung systems aren't made to take that kind of abuse."

Back in intensive care, Jean looks in on Mary again for a blow bottle treatment. She is in bed asleep. Her daughter is sitting in a chair next to the bed and looks up anxiously.

"This is the first time she's slept. She hasn't slept since midnight last night."

"That's OK," Jean says. "We won't bother her. I'll be back later." Jean stops by the nursing station and makes a note on her chart before heading downstairs for lunch.

The hospital cafeteria is crowded, but Jean finds her colleagues outside at a picnic table.

"Have you checked that croupette up in pediatrics?" Barb asks as she sits down.

"No, I was going to go up right after lunch, and do Bobbie at the same time. Then I'll go ahead with oxygen rounds."

"My husband has had a really big effect on my attitude toward patients," Jean says. "When I first went to work, if something personal went wrong, like if I came in a room and someone was crying I'd just go blank and say 'That's not my job.' My husband was a sociology major but he's working as a ward clerk now at a big hospital. He's already got a reputation there for knowing names, following up on patient needs. All the evidence shows that physical healing is enormously affected by psychological conditions, but they are too hard for most people to handle. People talk about not getting emotionally involved, in order to follow through on their work. Frankly, I find the opposite is true. Sometimes I have to force myself to make an identification in order to keep going.

With Emma for example... How do I avoid the temptation to cut the therapy short, not to do my best? What the hell. She's old. She's very unlikely to pull out of this thing. I have to think back to when my husband was in the hospital after an automobile accident, the treatment my mother got after her stroke, anything to remind me of the humanness of the situation. As far as supplying psychological needs... I've had very personal experience with that end of things. Both my kids were born by Caesarian section. I had a terrible time with depression, especially after the second one. I got excellent care medically, but there was no one to talk to... I really needed a sister, or a mother or someone around."

After lunch Jean goes back to the office briefly to pick up her charts and then rides to the fourth-floor pediatric ward. It has been newly remodeled with brightly colored rugs and graphics on the walls. A boy of seven is hurling himself along in a wheelchair after an older boy with a gun. Jean grabs the wheelchair as it flies by.

"You get ready for those blow bottles," she says in mock seriousness. "I'm comin' back to get ya', Bobbie." He grins.

The croupette Jean checks is a special oxygen tent for babies who have been suffering from the deep barky cough of croup. A mist, cooled by being passed through a large box-like container, enters a tent that resembles an oxygen tent.

"The best treatment for croup is cool damp air. It is a very frightening experience for the parents and child, and is often an emergency. It comes on suddenly and sometimes the windpipe can just swell up so badly that the child actually stops breathing.

"There, I made it right on time. The vaporizer box is all out of ice. Hi there, sweetheart." A blond-haired, healthy looking baby of about ten months grins eagerly. The child crawls over to the edge of the crib and whacks noisily on the clear plastic tent. "See, he looks just fine now. But it may come on suddenly again tonight. They almost always come in the emergency room at night." Jean goes down to the nursing station to get a bucket of ice. "Let's see if mother is here... oh yes, she's going back in. I like to have the mothers in the room when I put the ice in because it makes a pretty loud noise."

The mother, drawn and pale looking, is unzipping the tent to change the baby's diaper when Jean goes back into the room.

"OK, Baby, big noise now. There we go."

"We've been awfully lucky with illnesses with our kids, with both of us working," Jean says, as she goes down to Bobbie's room to get his blow bottles. "But even with that, I have a lot of bad feelings about having to work when they're little. They've always had good care, and socially they're very much at ease. But sometimes I think they get lonely. And I hate having to wake them up in the morning. It seems like they should be able to sleep if they want to."

Jean catches Bobbie in the hall and gets him through his blowing exercise quickly. He is recovering from abdominal surgery.

"This is one of the preventive things we do. To keep him using those lungs fully. With his stomach muscles being sore he has a tendency to splint his breathing or breathe shallow."

With her flip charts in hand, Jean makes the rounds of all the patients on oxygen. Most of them are in intensive care. She checks the connections on the hoses and the vapor bottles that are used to humidify the dry oxygen. She also checks the level on the bottles and records the meter readings for each patient for billing purposes.

"Leona," she greets a middle-aged woman sitting on the edge of a bed. "I thought you were going home today."

"Oh no," the woman smiles and shakes her head wearily. She has the short pinched breath of the emphysema patient. "They're waiting to do another blood gas test, and they can't find anyone who can get a vein anymore," she laughs.

"Well, you spoiled my record last week," Jean says. "I've never missed before."

"And Sue Binkley too. I asked for her especially. And the resident, Dr. Shepard, gave up. So they're waiting for Dr. Nelson. He won't be in for a bit yet. Oh, I just dread being stuck again."

"I guess you've just about run out of arterial sites." She checks the oxygen unit and makes a note in her books. "Are you off the oxygen?"

"No, not completely. But almost."

"Well, good luck, Leona."

"Thank you, dear."

"Poor Leona," Jean mutters back at the nursing station. "She's been in about five times since I've been here, I think. She still won't admit that she has emphysema. She keeps saying it's her ulcers. She's a very intelligent woman too. She's really very sick."

"Jean Tanner, 302." A voice comes over the intercom.

"Oh hell, I forgot to pick up my beeper. They like you to keep a beeper so the patients don't get bothered so much, but I keep forgetting."

"Yes?" she picks up the phone. "Oh, OK. How soon will they be ready? All right. Just two? OK. I'll be down in a bit."

Jean finishes writing in her charts. "I took a course last year on teaching CPR, Cardiopulmonary Resuscitation. We give it here for anyone on the staff who wants to take it, nurses, custodial people. Anyone. Then, when they feel they're ready, they take a written test and someone has to watch them go through the procedure to be certified. I think there are two people down there now, so I have to go do that."

Jean goes first to the office and gets her record writing done on the oxygen rounds and the pediatric treatments. In a classroom down the hall, two women are taking the written exam. In a corner of the room, Resusci-Ann, the CPR dummy model, is lying on a towel, and Baby is on a small table.

"Do you want to be certified for both Baby and Ann?"

The women nod.

"OK. Go ahead. Who's first?"

"I'll go," a woman in blue jeans and a red turtleneck shirt volunteers.

"OK. Now for the assisted, you do three cycles of fifteen and then she'll come in. OK? Go ahead."

"All right," the woman says. "Here goes. Annie! Annie! Are you all right?" She leans over the dummy's head, checks for obstructions, checks a pulse, then gives several breaths in her mouth.

"The pulse comes after the breaths," Jean says.

"OK. Shall I start again? . . . Annie! Annie! Are you all right?" When the woman starts the chest pushing motions Jean reminds her to slow down.

"Take the full time you're allowed. There's no sense in rushing. Take the time to think through what you're doing."

After the three cycles of breathing and pushing, the other woman steps up to the dummy.

"I know CPR," she says briskly. Then leans over to take over the mouth breathing, while the first woman continues the chest massage. After a few extra practices, Jean passes both women.

Jean still has a final round to go with Emma and a few more blow bottle treatments left. And always more paper work.

"As far as career planning goes . . . I think respiratory therapy is a place where some high-school courses are really helpful. Physics and biochemistry would be really helpful here in understanding the pulmonary system, how the gases respond in the body.

"For my own purposes, I don't really see this as being my career, in capital letters. I'm still interested in occupational therapy, just because it seems like a more total approach to care . . . it can even include parts of respiratory therapy. It involves training people with strokes, cancer patients, retarded people too, to care for themselves, to handle their life functions. I've already started taking some classes at the university. I could finish up in a year, but I think it would be too much of a strain on my home life. Ideally, I think I'd like to start my own therapy clinic, where I could really concentrate on my own priorities in health care.

"Oh, well," she shrugs cheerfully as she enters Emma's room again. "I'm only twenty-six. I figure I've got another twenty years to find a career."

SUMMARY

DUTIES: *Also called inhalation therapist. Treats cardiorespiratory problems. Uses respirators and positive pressure breathing machines to administer gases and medication to patients with emphysema, asthma and other problems. The respiratory therapist is often used in emergency situations with heart attack victims, drownings and drug overdoses.*

TRAINING: *Eighteen months to four years in an accredited program. Registry with the National Board of Respiratory Therapy requires graduation from an accepted program, sixty-two hours of college, one year of experience and passing an exam. The registry is not required for practice, but may help in getting a job. There are also respiratory technicians and aides who have less training. For more information, contact:*

> *American Association of Respiratory Therapy*
> *7411 Hines Place, Suite 101*
> *Dallas, Texas   75235*

SALARY: *$9,900 to start. Less for technicians and aides.*

10.

CLINICAL PSYCHOLOGIST

"You shouldn't have to be married to your job," Sue Larsen says, as she pulls through the gate of the city parking ramp. It is a cold day, grey clouds blending with the bleak city skyline. Sue drives fifteen miles into the city from the little farmhouse she rents in the country. "I've tried to avoid a conventional all-encompassing career. I've seen how unhealthy it can be. I make lots of outside commitments though. I have to fight a tendency to over-schedule myself."

Sue is a clinical psychologist. She is the one-person psychology department for the Methodist hospital in the city. She has resisted making it a full-time position. Instead, she is hired on an hourly basis and works three or four days a week. This leaves her time to keep some private patients. This morning, she is on her way to see private clients in the office she rents for herself. After circling the parking ramp several times, she finds an open space. Grabbing a briefcase from the back seat, she leaves the car and heads toward the stairs to the street.

Sue is a tall, attractive woman in her mid-thirties. She is casually dressed, her long dark hair tied back in a scarf. Her manner is one of gentleness combined with quiet curiosity.

Her office is on the third floor, between a beauty school and a law firm. She uses it only two or three times a week. It is sparsely furnished—a phone, a couch, two chairs, carpeted floors. Piles of large cushions in the corner can be used for group therapy.

"This morning, I'm doing a 'mediation' with a couple. It's a more or less formal method of problem solving. The method is outlined in advance. You really need a plan. With couples, things easily break down into a screaming fight. Of course, they don't need me to do that. They can do that on their own time."

There is a tentative knock on the door and a man and woman step in. They are in their late twenties. They are both wearing blue jeans. The man shuffles a bit and turns his fists in the pockets of his green parka. The woman smiles and brushes her hair behind her ear.

"Hi, I'm Sue Larsen." Sue gets up from the couch and goes to greet them. "You are Tom and Laura?" They nod. "Well. Come in. You can put your coats on the floor. We don't seem to have any hangers here." Tom and Laura remove their coats, exchanging quick glances at each other. "Do you have any preference for sitting? We've got two chairs, or you can sit on the floor."

"The chairs are fine," Tom says. Laura and Tom seat themselves in two wooden captain's chairs that face the couch.

Sue sits down at one end of the couch. She puts a blank piece of paper in a clip board and writes "Tom and Laura" at the top.

"Did we talk about payment when you spoke to me earlier?"

"Yeah. We said thirty-five."

"Oh, we did. OK. I couldn't remember. I always like to check to make sure there's no misunderstanding."

"Well, I'm only working part time now so . . . "

"That's fine. Just so we agree." Sue re-ties the scarf in her hair. "Before we get into the actual mediation, I think we should talk about any hang-ups you might have about coming into therapy. If there is anything about me you don't like or might have heard, it would be good to bring it up now. It could get in our way later."

"Well, I work at the hospital now," Laura says quietly. "I saw a woman do a mediation session with a couple as a demonstration. I thought it was good. It might really help us."

"How about you, Tom?" Sue asks.

"No," Tom shrugs. "I don't have any problems really." Laura looks at him with raised eyebrows.

"What about this morning . . . what you said?"

"That was nothing," Tom says sternly. "I just made an off-the-cuff remark about therapists. But I didn't mean it and I really don't think it should be brought up now."

"OK. That's up to you," Sue says. "The sessions usually take about two hours. If we follow the patterns that we set up, we should get somewhere in that time. We start out by having you air some of the resentments and paranoias you have about the other person. After the resentments and paranoias, we'll get into some of the good things you have to say about each other. I use 'paranoias' to refer to fears or suspicions you may have about the other person. These fears are usually exaggerated but have some little grain of truth that is important to deal with. The final part will be expressing what you would consider 100 percent satisfaction from the mediation. Then we can start working toward a compromise, a kind of contract that will bring you some of that. Are you married, by the way?"

"No," Laura says. "We've been living together for two years. I guess that's the core of the problem right now . . . trying to reach a decision about getting married."

"I see. As we get into the resentments and paranoias, there are some rules to follow. First you have to find out if the other person wants to hear the paranoia or resentment. You need to get permission. When you state your resentments, try to make them as specific as possible. Instead of saying 'You're always burping,' say 'Last Sunday when you were at so and so's house, you burped out loud and it really embarrassed me.' With resentments, the other person doesn't need to comment. With the paranoias there is usually some grain of truth in the feelings. When people tell you 'Oh that's just not true,' it can make you feel crazy. So it's important for the other person to verify that grain of truth. Who wants to start? Laura, do you have a resentment you'd like to get out?"

"Well, yeah, I guess I feel . . . "

"Check it out with Tom first."

"Tom, can I tell you a resentment I have?"

"Yes. I'm a little uptight that you might say something that would seem too personal to me. But, I guess it's OK. Yeah, go ahead."

"Well, this is something we've talked about before. It's nothing new, but I do . . . I have to resent your unwillingness to decide about marriage. I mean, one way or the other. It doesn't seem fair."

"I know, Laura. I'm doing the best I can."

"OK," Sue interrupts gently. "That's OK. You don't need to answer a resentment. Just leave it. We'll go on from here. How about you, Tom? Do you have a resentment or paranoia?"

"Yeah, I do have a paranoia. I have a lot!" he laughs. "But I guess one would be . . . " He stops himself. "Do you want to hear this, Laura?" She nods. "Well, it's a fear about myself in a way. You see," He turns to Sue. "We . . . I mean Laura, has set up a kind of deadline of March 1. We decide then to get married or split. I don't blame her for it. I understand. But I guess my fear is . . . the decision seems impossible to me, even though it's six months away. My first marriage was so bad. I just don't know if I can do it again. Anyway, my fear is that if I decide I can't marry her she'll think it's because I don't love her. That wouldn't be true, but I'm afraid she wouldn't understand that."

"Do you want to validate the truth in that, Laura?" Sue says.

"Well." She glances between Sue and Tom. "I want to marry Tom, there's no doubt about that. But I know him well enough now to know he loves me. Splitting up would be tough . . . but I've been through it before. I'm not that weak. Fear of hurting me is certainly no reason to get married."

Sue follows Laura and Tom through the catalogue of resentments and fears in their lives together: his motorcycle, her dependence, his brooding silences, her parents. Tom and Laura become more articulate as they progress. It is obvious they have discussed most of the subjects before, but the formal setting seems to take some of the emotional burden away. They smile frequently at their own exaggerations. They seem to like each other.

"Well," Sue glances at her watch. "I think we're making some progress, but we are running out of time. Do you want to negotiate for another half hour, or try to make an appointment for some other time?"

Tom and Laura debate briefly about their different work schedules. They decide to go on for a half hour now.

"Well, just to summarize, I'd like to tell you what I see developing," Sue says, "so we can move toward negotiating some kind of compromise. Tom is the one who is reluctant about marriage and Laura, you seem to feel pretty positive about it. I think it would be helpful to outline the positive and negative feelings you've come up with . . . what marriage means to you. How about you, Laura?"

"Well, it's a promise, a commitment to staying together, to being a life partner. And the possibility of having kids someday. It's a promise. And for me right now, the social pressure is great. I mean, to get married."

"Yes, social pressure is real," Sue says. "Of course, I think there is more acceptance today of alternative arrangements."

"It's not our friends that are pushing, it's the parents. Both sets. They both live in the city. They really want us to get married."

"Tom, how about you? Do you want to go over some of the negative things you see in marriage?"

"It changes things. I don't care what other people say. No matter how close you are to being married, living together is different. The dependence would bother me, but more than that, it's just being seen by your friends as a married man. It really changes your friendships ... limits them. I'm not talking about other women, other sexual relationships. I just mean friendships. People treat you differently."

Sue then moves toward having Tom and Laura express 100 percent of what they would like to get out of the mediation session.

"I want you to extend yourselves," Sue says. "Be greedy. Sometimes people compromise inside before they start talking. It's better to say what your real dreams are, and work from there." There is a long pause.

"Peace of mind," Tom says finally, and smiles at Laura.

By the end of the session, it is almost twelve-thirty. Sue goes into a health food deli around the corner from her office for a quick sandwich.

"I like most of my clients," Sue says. "Tom and Laura were easy to like. They had about the shortest list of resentments I've ever had in a mediation with a couple. But doing therapy with the few people you don't like is really a drag."

"The avocados aren't ripe," the waitress apologizes, setting down Sue's sandwich. "I added alfalfa sprouts instead." Sue nods her approval.

"I've become involved with what is known now as radical therapy," Sue explains. "For me this is basically just seeing people's problems in a social context instead of as isolated nuttiness. For example ... I have a housewife who comes in complaining of severe depression, fatigue, anxiety. She tells me about her day ... the strenuous life she leads for her husband and her children. I say, 'What do you do for yourself?' She says, 'Nothing ... there isn't time.' She lives totally for the approval of her family. Her depression isn't any more bizarre than a cold someone catches in a drafty house. The problem is getting her to try some other patterns."

After lunch, Sue moves on to the hospital.

"There is someone else who works as a part-time psychologist here. We're also in the process of hiring someone to do the psychological testing. I spend a fair amount of time doing that now ... giving various tests to stroke and accident patients to determine the extent of brain damage. The rest of my case load is referrals from doctors, usually stroke patients or patients who have been depressed or difficult."

Sue's office in the hospital is on the fifth floor. She sifts through the patient records lying on a table by her desk and pulls one out.

"This patient I'm going to see now is a referral from the Speech and Language Pathology and Audiology department in the hospital. He was being seen as an outpatient for a stuttering problem, but the therapist thought he could use some extra attention. He's very withdrawn. I'm trying to work on getting him to go out a little ... meet people. He lives by himself in a boarding house." The phone on Sue's desk rings. "Yes? Hi Ann ... I'm going to see Frank now. That'll take an hour. I'll meet you in your office right after that ... OK."

"Ann is the head of the speech clinic," Sue explains as she takes the elevator down to the outpatient clinic. "We're putting a slide show together for her to take to a convention next week. It's about using radical therapy in speech work."

Frank Jones is seated in a chair in the waiting room. He is short with a round face and sandy hair and freckles. He looks younger than his thirty years. He stands, smiling, when he sees Sue. His arms are filled with books. Sue greets him with a smile, too.

"I see you've brought your library," Sue says softly.

"I w-w-w-w-." Frank pauses, his face pinched with effort, then starts again. "I went to the library before I came here."

"Well, let's go down the hall. I think there's an empty room down here. Yes, there is."

The room has two office desks and two swivel chairs. There are boxes of toys on the floor and charts on the walls that are used with children during therapy. Sue and Frank seat themselves in the swivel chairs facing one another. Frank fingers his books as Sue takes out a clip board and reaches for a pen. Sue waits a few seconds. Frank fingers his books some more. After a few more moments of silence, Sue begins.

"Well, how have things been going this week, Frank?"

"Oh, f-f-f-f-. Oh f-f-f-f-fine." Frank says. "Fine. I went to class and worked. The usual."

"Nothing special happened?"

"Oh, I got my psych test back. I got a C+. I was h-h-h-h-h-. I was happy about that."

"That sounds great." Sue pauses. "The last time we met we talked about setting goals for doing more socially. Have you done any thinking about that?"

"Well, at school I've no-no-no . . . " Frank pauses. "I've no-no-noticed a few people from classes around . . . I can talk to them."

"You're getting to know some people in your classes?"

"Well, some." There is a lengthy pause. "There was one g-g-g-girl in my psych class. She came over when I was having a Coke and talked. Before class."

"That sounds good. How did you feel talking to her? Were you comfortable?"

"Yes, I felt comfortable. B-b-b-b. B-b-ut it's not a big thing."

"Well, no. But you have to start with small things. The more comfortable you get in these situations, the easier it will be to make friends."

"I've been reading a lot," Frank smiles.

"You always read a lot," Sue says, looking over Frank's books. "*Space Colonies*?"

"Yes. I believe this may h-h-h-happen soon. That we can send people into space to colonize."

"Do you?"

"I wrote my senator about it."

"About what?"

"About support for the space program."

"Let's talk about some goals we could set for you, Frank. I'd like to set up something concrete for next week. Do you have any ideas?"

Frank shrugs. "Not really. Nothing special."

"Do you play any games, or sports?"

"I play chess sometimes. I played w-w-w-w-w. I played with someone after class last week."

"You enjoyed it?"

"Yes. He beat me, though."

"Well. That's OK. It will be easier for you to socialize, I think, if you plan something to do, so you don't have to worry about what you're going to say."

"Yes, that would be nice."

"How many times do you think you'd like to play chess this week?"

"Oh, m-m-m-m. Maybe three. Maybe three."

"Good. I'll write that down."

At the end of the hour, Sue walks toward the lobby with Frank. She says good-bye to him and turns toward the speech and hearing office.

"Frank was very calm today," Sue says. "He leads a lonely life. All the books on space and stuff are not a joke for him. I think he really feels he would be more at home in a space colony. He feels like an alien here. I don't go in and tell him he's crazy to think he's an alien. There is a grain of truth in his feeling. He's been shuffled around schools and family. I've tried to emphasize for him the possibility of finding a colony on this earth . . . a group of people who have shared interests. It's what we're all looking for."

Ann is waiting for Sue in her office. She has a stack of slides on her desk and a pile of papers.

"How did Frank do with you today?" Ann asks.

"It's hard to tell. He seems to be making progress. He talks about making some social contacts. It's hard to tell how much he really does."

"I know what you mean. I had speech therapy with him this morning. He talks about practicing his speech techniques . . . it's hard to say."

"What's going on here?" Sue points to the slides.

"I want you to take a look at the slides and then go over the script with me. It's going to be on an automatic slide projector and tape deal. I'll just set it up in the display area at the convention. Marcia and Don said they'd come in and record the script with us in half an hour. Do you have the time?"

"Yes. I have an appointment at four. It shouldn't take that long."

The first slide has the title of the presentation: "Power and Prejudice in Clinical Practice."

CLINICAL PSYCHOLOGIST

"This shows some of the basics of radical therapy applied to speech therapy," Sue explains. "I guess I got Ann interested in it. We're showing just one aspect in this show ... it's about rescuing. Rescuing is when a therapist takes over all the responsibility for what happens in therapy. In radical therapy, the clinician and the client are supposed to be in a contract situation ... sharing the responsibility fifty-fifty. It leads to less guilt and frustration for the therapist and less resentment in the client."

It is almost four o'clock by the time Sue and the others finish recording the soundtrack for the slide show. Sue climbs the five flights of stairs to her office. From the back of her file cabinet she pulls out a box with materials for the MMPI test, the Minnesota Multiphasic Personality Inventory, and heads upstairs.

"This next client is a teenager who's up in the psychiatric ward. I don't know exactly why he needs the evaluation. His psychiatrist has really gotten into testing recently. My contact with the doctors is generally on the negative side. We have some basic philosophical differences. I believe that patients should know as much about their illness and treatment as possible. Most doctors, however, don't feel this way. They want to hold all the cards. I think that's a bad situation for the patient. The doctors are still taught that their authority is supreme. They don't seem to have much respect for the patients' rights or opinions."

Sue goes to the nursing station on the psychiatric ward and asks a nurse to page Larry McDonald.

"This boy is sixteen ... on withdrawal from drugs. He was picked up on a B and E, breaking and entering, a couple of times. This stay in the hospital is an attempt to get him stabilized and to do some evaluation before he has to go to court."

Larry shuffles down the hall from his room. He is wearing faded blue jeans and a flannel shirt. His hair is long, but clean and neatly combed.

"Hi," he greets Sue quietly in the hall, then follows her to an empty room. They sit on opposite sides of a desk. The last light from the grey day outside filters through a small dirty window. Larry sits with his legs stretched out in front, chewing solemnly on a fingernail.

"How are things going, Larry?" Sue asks, unpacking materials from the test box. "I meant to come see you yesterday, but we had a last minute meeting."

"Things are goin' pretty good," Larry says. "I thought it would be grim here, but I've made some friends. It's all right."

"Did you go out on pass?"

"Yeah. I went home Saturday to visit my mom."

"How long have you been out of school, Larry?"

"I quit when I was fourteen. Two years ago."

"Why did you quit?"

"I thought it would be neat to get out and work and have money. I was on drugs all the time in school anyway. I couldn't concentrate or nothin'. It was a waste. I think I could go back now though."

"Why is that?"

"It just wasn't that great bein' out. I spent all my money on drugs ... I only worked for four months anyway. There wasn't much work. I was all burned out. My mom was gettin' on my ass all the time. We'd fight a lot."

"Did you usually fight?"

"No. I never used to fight with her. I was always pretty happy ... smiled at everyone. But things got bad. I had some bad trips and was just sittin' around all the time. I got kind of nasty. I'm almost glad I got that B and E."

"Why is that?"

" 'Cause I think I can get some help now. Get off drugs. I haven't had anything since I been in here. It's not too bad. This weekend will be the big test, 'cause I'm goin' home for the whole weekend."

"Well, I hope you can make it," Sue says. "I've got to do some testing now, to see how we might be able to help you. In this first section, I'm going to say some words ... "

Sue and Larry work together for about half an hour. As Sue leaves the ward, she checks with the nurse to make sure she can see Larry the next day to finish.

"I don't see any possibility of brain damage or anything like that," Sue says. "You don't like to be cynical, but with a street-wise kid like that, the remorse and wanting to go back to school ... well, it's pretty heavy for one week of drying out. You have to ask whether it's something he wants the judge to see on his report."

Sue meets Ann and her husband on the way out of the hospital and they head out for a pizza. Sue still has a meeting to attend this evening before she heads home.

"I'm helping some friends get a men's center started at the college here in town," Sue explains. "If we get a certain number of students involved, we can get a meeting place and funding from the school. There are a lot of personal skills men haven't learned because of sexism . . . being in touch with emotions, knowing how to relate to children, to help people. They asked me to help because I've worked on getting a women's center started."

After dinner, Sue finds her way to the meeting room in the student union. She is the only woman at the meeting. She sits quietly, and answers occasional questions about funding, how to hold an open-house and what kinds of programs are successful.

By the time the organizational meeting is over, it is almost ten o'clock. Sue is finally heading for home.

"I'm drawn more and more to looking at the social environment of people with psychological problems. What society asks of people isn't always healthy for them. I guess the best example I can think of is a patient I had a while ago. He was a social worker . . . a very dynamic and committed and success-oriented man. He wanted to be the best. He took on every extra responsibility he could. He worked constantly.

"He came in complaining of migraine headaches, stomach problems, times where he would be so fatigued he would pull his car over and fall asleep at the wheel. I talked to him about the whole male-success thing, how dangerous it was . . . heart attacks, high blood pressure. It wasn't unlike the housewife's problem. He wasn't doing anything to look out for himself. He was living for the eyes of the world.

"I had been seeing him for a while on a weekly basis. I don't know how much I was getting through to him. But fate stepped in for me. He came in one day looking grim as hell. He told me one of his colleagues had died of a heart attack . . . the most well-respected and popular worker in the department, a man who had literally worked his heart out. The day after the funeral my client went into the office. No one mentioned the departed. No one talked about him or wept or anything. There wasn't anything left of his work. Everything went on without him." Sue pauses. "It was pretty powerful therapy."

Sue stifles a yawn as she turns off the highway toward her home.

"Anyway, work is a strange thing. Nothing seems to panic people more than free time. It's a problem I wrestle with myself."

SUMMARY

DUTIES: *Clinical psychologists generally work in mental hospitals or clinics. Sometimes they see private patients as well. They deal with problems of the mentally ill and emotionally disturbed. They also help deal with the emotional impact of injury or disease in the hospital. They interview patients, give diagnostic tests and do individual, family and group therapy.*

TRAINING: *A Ph.D is generally needed for work in clinical psychology. This means three to five years of training after the college BA. One of these years is usually an internship in a hospital or clinic. For more information, contact:*

> *American Psychological Association*
> *1200 17th Street NW*
> *Washington, D.C. 20036*

SALARY: *Starting salary for a clinical psychologist with a Ph.D averages $16,500. Experienced clinical psychologists in private practice can earn $38,000 or more.*

RELATED OCCUPATIONS

MUSIC THERAPIST

DUTIES: *Music therapists use music and musical activities to assist in therapy goals. As a member of a treatment team, the music therapist aids in the analysis of the patient's problem and plans specific hospital activities. Music therapists work primarily in psychiatric hospitals and mental health centers, but also work in some general hospital wards, nursing homes and schools for the handicapped.*

TRAINING: *Music therapy usually requires a BA in the field. This is offered at some universities now. The training consists of a combination of music and psychology. To be registered, the therapist must have a six-month internship. For more information, contact:*

> *National Association of Music Therapy*
> *P.O. Box 610*
> *Lawrence, Kansas   66044*

SALARY: *$10,000 to start.*

DIETETIC TECHNICIAN

DUTIES: *The dietetic technician works under a registered hospital dietician in planning menus for patients, instructing outpatients, such as diabetics, in proper diet, and planning nutrition courses for patients and hospital personnel.*

TRAINING: *A two-year associate degree program at a university or community college, and experience under a registered dietician are required. For more information, contact:*

> *American Dietetic Association*
> *620 North Michigan Avenue*
> *Chicago, Illinois   10011*

SALARY: *$9,000 to start.*

ELECTROENCEPHALOGRAPHIC TECHNICIAN

DUTIES: *This technician uses a machine called an electroencephalograph to record the brain activity of a patient. The technician observes the patient's behavior, makes notes during the recording and is alert for signs of an emergency condition. The EEG technician has to have control of the patient during the recording time.*

TRAINING: *Until recently, EEG technicians were trained on the job with just a high-school degree. Formal training programs are now in existence and are probably the wave of the future. There are now two-year technologist programs and six-month technician programs at universities and community colleges. For more information, contact:*

American Society of Electroencephalographic Technologists
University of Iowa
Division of Electroencephalography and Neurophysiology
500 Newton Road
Iowa City, Iowa 52242

SALARY: *$7,800 to start. Experienced technologists may earn up to $20,000.*

NUCLEAR MEDICAL PSYCHOLOGIST

DUTIES: *Nuclear medical technologists use radioactive materials in the diagnosis and treatment of malignant disease. They operate equipment such as scintillation detectors and scanners, and prepare radioactive isotopes for administration to patients. They assist the physician in administering the isotopes. They also help the patient get situated and explain the nature of the tests and treatments to the patient.*

TRAINING: *The length of training varies from one year to three years beyond high school. Programs are available in hospitals, junior colleges and universities. For more information, contact:*

American Society of Radiologic Technologists
645 North Michigan Avenue, Suite 836
Chicago, Illinois 60611

SALARIES: *$10,000–12,000 to start.*

PROSTHETIST-ORTHOTIST

DUTIES: *The Prosthetist-Orthotist writes specifications for and fits artificial limbs, braces and appliances for body deformities, as prescribed by a physician or other medical personnel. S/he examines the body for bumps or bruises that might affect the fit. Then s/he measures the limb or deformity to be fitted. The appliance is made by an orthopedic appliance and limb technician. The prosthetist-orthotist fits the appliance and instructs the patient in its use. If the person specializes in making limbs, s/he is called a prosthetist. If s/he specializes in braces and support appliances, s/he may be an orthotist.*

TRAINING: *Training requirements are in the process of changing. High-school graduation with a four-year informal apprenticeship is still possible. Some colleges have begun four-year programs leading to a BS in the area. Others enter the field with a BA and a six-to-ten-week course in biomechanics as it relates to orthotic and prosthetic appliances. It is predicted that by 1980 a BS will be needed to enter this field. For more information, contact:*

American Orthotics-Prosthetics Association
919 18th Street NW
Washington, D.C. 20006

SALARY: *$9,000 starting for those with a BA.*

OCCUPATIONAL THERAPIST

DUTIES: *The occupational therapist conducts programs in hospitals or other institutions to rehabilitate the physically or mentally handicapped. Manual arts and crafts, prevocational and homemaking skills, as well as educational, recreational and social activities are taught to adjust the patient to her/his handicap. The occupational therapist evaluates the patient's progress and establishes goals that are appropriate. This may include the gradual expansion of activities for a stroke patient, or assisting the recent surgical patient in adjusting to her/his confinement.*

TRAINING: *Many four-year colleges now offer a BA in occupational therapy. The occupational therapist makes use of aides and technicians who require less training. For more information, contact:*

> American Occupational Therapy Association
> 250 West 57th Street
> New York, New York   10017

SALARY: *$9,000–12,000 to start. Administrators may earn up to $30,000.*

RADIOLOGIC TECHNOLOGIST (X-RAY TECHNOLOGIST)

DUTIES: *The radiologic technologist operates X-ray machines to take pictures of internal organs and bones. The technologist may also prepare the barium salts that are taken to make certain organs show up on the X-ray picture. The technologist assists the patient in positioning her/himself correctly for the picture. S/he is also responsible for strict safety procedures so that neither s/he nor the patient is exposed to excessive radiation.*

TRAINING: *Training varies from two-year programs to community college programs to four-year BA programs. The BA will probably not give a person a higher starting salary, but it will afford greater opportunity for advancement. For more information, contact:*

> American Society of Radiologic Technologists
> 500 North Michigan Avenue, Suite 836
> Chicago, Illinois   60611

SALARY: *$9,000 to start.*

PHYSICAL THERAPIST

DUTIES: *The physical therapist organizes and conducts medically prescribed programs in hospitals, residential institutions and public health agencies. S/he plans physical therapy programs for each patient, using exercise, massage, heat, water, light and electrical treatments. S/he does diagnostic tests on muscle, nerve and joint functions. S/he educates patients in postural control and exercise that can be continued after hospital stays. S/he is in charge of keeping the therapy area supplied with necessary equipment.*

TRAINING: *The physical therapist needs a BS in the field plus a four-month internship. Most states now require a licensing examination in order to practice. For more information, contact:*

American Physical Therapy Association
1740 Broadway
New York, New York   10019

SALARY: *$9,600–16,000, depending on experience and location.*

ENVIRONMENTAL HEALTH TECHNICIAN

DUTIES: *The environmental health technician assists the sanitarian in getting people to conform to state and federal laws concerning water, purity, garbage and sewage disposal. The environmental health technician is usually employed in a waste water treatment plant, but is also used in other enforcement areas.*

TRAINING: *The two-year associate arts degree is the accepted training for environmental health technicians. Some junior colleges have training programs now and more are developing. For more information, contact:*

National Environmental Health Association
1200 Lincoln Street, Suite 704
Denver, Colorado   80203

SALARY: *$9,000–11,000 to start.*

DENTAL LABORATORY TECHNICIAN

DUTIES: *The dental lab technician constructs and repairs dentures, bridges, crowns and inlays according to the dentist's prescription. Techniques used include encasing wax dentures in plastic or plaster and melting out the wax to inject plastic inside. Porcelain crowns may be shaped by hand and then glazed over. Generalists are involved in all areas. It is also possible to work in one area only, such as the crown and bridge, or the bite block.*

TRAINING: *One to two years of training after high school, usually in a junior college or technical school. The technician then works three to four years before taking the certifying exam. For more information, contact:*

National Association of Certified Dental Labs
1230 Massachusetts Ave NW
Washington, D.C.   20005

SALARY: *$7,500 to start. May rise to $15,000 with experience.*

MEDICAL RECORDS TECHNICIAN

DUTIES: *The medical records technician prepares reports, and codes diseases and operations by established patterns. S/he must check all sections of a patient's file for missing information, and must find files when requested. The medical record is a critical element in the treatment of a patient. The technician is often called on to take records to court and represent the hospital when records have been subpoenaed. The medical records technician may also be asked to take minutes at staff meetings and keep them on file.*

TRAINING: *High-school graduation plus graduation from a school of medical records technicians at a hospital or technical school. A home-study course is also available for medical records technicians. For more information, contact:*

> American Medical Records Association
> 875 North Michigan Avenue, Suite 1850
> Chicago, Illinois 60611

SALARY: *Salaries vary greatly, ranging from $5,000 in the southern states to $11,000 in New York City.*

CYTOTECHNOLOGIST

DUTIES: *The cytotechnologist is involved with the laboratory examination of cells. S/he stains, mounts, and examines cells for evidence of cancer and other disease conditions. S/he takes body materials, such as blood, scrapings and exudants. The cells are separated in centrifuges. A specimen is then placed on a slide, put in fixative and stained to make certain parts stand out. The cytotechnologist classifies the condition of cells according to established standards ranging from normal to abnormal. Questionable slides are shown to the pathologist. The cytotechnologist records results of all tests performed, and maintains the records for the laboratory.*

TRAINING: *The cytotechnologist needs two years of college, with an emphasis on biology and chemistry, plus a year in a school of cytotechnology. For more information, contact:*

> American Society of Medical Technologists
> Herman Professional Building, Suite 25
> Houston, Texas 77025

SALARY: *$9,200 to start.*

AUDIOMETRIST

DUTIES: *The audiometrist administers hearing tests to adults and children for diagnosis and possible rehabilitation. The tests are prescribed by a physician or an audiologist. The audiometrist interviews the patient and explains the tests to her/him. S/he puts the earphones on the patient, outlines the procedures and records the patient's responses. Records are kept which are used by the audiologist or physician in diagnosis.*

TRAINING: *The audiometrist needs a BA in Speech and Hearing. For more information, contact:*

> *The American Speech and Hearing Association*
> *1001 Connecticut Avenue, NW*
> *Washington, D.C. 20036*

SALARY: *$9,000 to start. May rise to $13,000 with experience.*

the organizers

Fifty years ago most hospitals were not much different from a boarding home. Now many are large, complex institutions with multi-million dollar annual budgets and, sometimes, million dollar deficits. As the health-care system has become more complex, there has been an increasing demand for individuals with administrative skills, people who can hold things together and make them work. Most of those who have administrative positions in the health system have no formal training for such work. They have started out as physicians, nurses, pharmacists, and such, and have eventually found themselves in supervisory or administrative positions. Some enjoy this work and see it as an opportunity; others find it just an added headache and would prefer, on many days, to return to the clinical duties they were trained for. It is only recently that administrators have begun to be formally trained for such roles. Increasingly, administrative positions are being reserved for those who have had some formal preparation.

There is a variety of such positions available. Boarding homes, nursing homes, medical groups and acute care hospitals require administrators. In the larger, more complex institutions there are many specialized administrative jobs that need to be done, such as medical records, financial management, service unit management and personnel administration. In addition, all the pieces of the health system have to be tied together in some way so that they can work most effectively. Health planners work at this. So do those who are responsible for administering health insurance plans.

In the following three chapters you will meet three people who work to make sure that people get what they need from our increasingly complex health-care system. The first is a ward clerk in a community hospital. She is responsible for making sure that patients on her floor get the lab tests, diets, drugs and therapy they need. The second runs a small, unlicensed boarding home. Her residents have many chronic illness problems and they need a supervised living arrangement. The third is the administrator of a large urban teaching hospital. He is responsible for balancing the conflicting needs of patients and the community with the limited amount of money he has to do the job. All three share the common goal of making things work.

11

WARD CLERK

Mary Ann Williams drives through the gate at the hospital employee parking lot at eight-fifteen. She's early, so she takes her time walking to the entrance. Eastern Community Hospital rises six stories above the row houses that surround it. The bright brick walls make the hospital stand out even more from its faded, cluttered surroundings.

"Hi, Janet. How was the vacation?" Mary Ann asks. She stops to chat with a friend who is a licensed practical nurse on another floor of the hospital. They arrange to have lunch together in the hospital cafeteria.

The breakfast trays are just being picked up as she gets off the elevator on her floor. It is a long narrow corridor with double rooms along each side. The "Today Show" flickers silently on the color television set inside one of the rooms. There are twenty-six patients on floor 4B.

"We get all kinds ... medical, surgical ... some just waiting to get into a nursing home," Mary Ann says, as she glances down the corridor.

A white-haired woman passes in a grey hospital bathrobe. She walks slowly, wincing with each step.

"Hi, Mrs. Ferguson. Feeling better?"

The woman smiles and nods.

The nursing station is squeezed into the side of the hall, halfway down the corridor. There is a long high counter on the front, and a desk level counter behind with three swivel chairs. Several nurses are standing at the counter talking. They exchange greetings with Mary Ann and she gets down to work.

Since it's still quiet on the floor, she begins by updating the patient records. The morning temperature, pulse and blood pressure readings have to be transcribed from the floor record sheet into each patient's record. She works quickly, pulling the metal patient record folders from the rack behind her and adding the new readings to the broken line graphs in the folders.

As she does this, she continues to chat with the nurses. Another joins them. They talk about a patient who was sent to the intensive care unit earlier that morning, then about last night's baseball game. Mary Ann's blue zippered uniform distinguishes her from the nurses in their white uniforms but she's treated as an equal. They enjoy her company. She's outgoing, bouncy, with an opinion on any topic. They also know they can count on her.

"Mary Ann is the most important person on this unit," one of the nurses says. "We can always replace a nurse if one is sick, but not Mary Ann. We won't allow her to take any sick days."

"Thanks," Mary Ann laughs.

Mary Ann's job includes answering the telephone, scheduling the tests, ordering the medications and other supplies, transcribing physician orders for patients into the nursing Cardex, organizing new charts, arranging transportation for patients, arranging for changes in a patient's diet, arranging clinic appointments, scheduling physician consultations that are ordered and a number of other things. She plays a part in almost everything that happens on the floor.

"I was in the college preparatory track in high school. By the time I was a senior I was sure of only one thing—I didn't want to go to school any more—at least not for a while. During my senior year I helped out on the weekends as a desk clerk. Right after I graduated, a full-time job opened up and I took it. I've been working here now for four years. I was really scared at first. There was so much I didn't know and everybody seemed to take it for granted that I knew everything. I think it would probably be helpful for a person taking a job like this to have a course in medical technology. Courses like that are taught in junior colleges and high schools. They teach you about the different kinds of terminology that are used. It's a whole different language. Anyway, it took me at least six months to get the hang of it. I feel comfortable and in control now except when things get very busy."

The phone rings.

"4B, Desk Clerk. Yup. OK."

WARD CLERK

Mary Ann writes something on the back of an old form, then hangs up. She pulls out a yellow form from a wooden rack attached to the wall. Altogether there are thirty-two different forms that Mary Ann works with. This one is for entering a verbal laboratory report into a patient's record. In this case, a blood count has been done.

"The lab only phones up the stuff that's really important to have right away." Mary Ann explains. "I take the message and make sure it gets in the patient's record. The routine lab reports are sent up by messenger. I replace the verbal report with the written one when it gets up here."

The forms Mary Ann works with fall into three general categories. One set of forms is used for ordering various tests and procedures. These include forms for X rays, hematology, transfusions, urinanalysis, microbiology and special therapy. They are envelope size and have two carbon copies. The original is kept as a part of the patient's record, one copy goes to the department providing the services and a third copy is used by the billing department to determine how much a patient will be charged for her or his visit to the hospital.

Another set of forms is used directly by the nursing staff to guide the care they give patients. There are two of these forms. One is a card-sized form that includes the nursing care plan for a particular patient. Mary Ann transcribes most of the information from the patient record to the card and updates it each day. These cards are kept in a portable metal folder stored on the counter for easy reference by the nurses. Another card, the same size, is a record of medications that should be given each patient. Mary Ann transcribes this information from the form the doctor fills out and orders the medication. The doctor's original order is kept in the medical record. The medication cards are kept in a similar long metal folder on the medication cart. The nurses wheel the cart down the hallway when they dispense the medications. Many patients receive more than five different medications during a given day.

The final set of forms is a part of the permanent patient record kept in the metal folders behind the desk. The permanent patient record includes information from the admission interview given by a nurse. The history and physical examination form completed by the patient's physician, nursing notes, physician completed progress notes, the medication administration record completed by the nurse, physician order forms, temperature, pulse and blood pressure charts, laboratory reports and a final discharge summary written by the physician are included as well. After a person is discharged, Mary Ann makes sure everything is complete and in order and sends it back to the records department.

She looks at something in one of the records. Puzzled, she shows it to one of the nurses.

"Yeah. Better check it out," the nurse says.

She dials a number and then winces. "I swear, I spend all of my time on the telephone and most of the time I'm on hold."

"Oh. Hello, Dr. Baker. I wanted to check on why they had cut out the insulin on a patient we have here and then increased it... Any X rays?... Yeah, let's see, he had a BE (Barium Enema X ray) this morning."

The nurse nods.

"OK, that's probably it. Thanks."

Another nurse empties pills from the medication cart into a bag and puts them on the counter next to Mary Ann.

"I get this job," says Mary Ann. "Because nobody else wants it." She takes the pills out of the bag and begins counting them. There are eight different medications.

"This patient has been discharged," Mary Ann explains. "We take the pills he didn't use, ship them back to the pharmacy and credit his account."

A man with long white hair walks past the nursing station. There is a nurse at each elbow. They help carry the two IV bottles which have tubes taped to the man's arms.

"You're looking good, Mr. Ross," Mary Ann says.

"Oh, I'm fine," Mr. Ross answers. His voice quavers.

"Hey, Mr. Ross," another nurse chips in. "Look, your hair is longer than mine. You need to have it cut." She pulls at a lock of the man's hair and smiles at him.

"Oh, I'm fine," Mr. Ross says again. He continues his slow pace down the corridor, not seeming to have heard. Mary Ann returns to her pill counting.

"As you can see," Mary Ann says, "I take care of a lot of the details. When someone dies on this floor, I notify information.

They contact the relatives. They're not allowed to tell them the person has died, they just tell them to come to the hospital. I order the stuff from central supply to wrap the body, and I try to make sure there's someone on the floor to head off the relatives so that they don't walk in while the body is being prepared. I notify the patient's doctor and the nursing office. We try to get the physician in charge of the case or one of the other physicians to break the news to the relatives. Father Sullivan is also very helpful in talking to the relatives."

Death, for Mary Ann, is part of the routine. She discusses it in the same matter-of-fact way she does the other details of her job.

Three physicians arrive at the nursing station. Mary Ann hands each several medical charts without a word being spoken between them.

"I follow around after the doctors and pick up after them," she says. "I've got to make sure that their orders are transcribed into the Cardex." She points to a set of flip folders on the edge of the desk. "This is used for the nurses to carry out treatment plans. The drug prescriptions have to be entered into a separate Cardex and put on the drug cart. Then I have to follow up and schedule the various laboratory tests and X rays and other therapeutic procedures they want performed.

"One thing that gets kind of irritating at times is the lack of communication. The physicians and the nurses expect a lot of things from you but they usually don't tell you what they are. We get only occasional supervision. You know, most of our work is within standard guidelines and procedures. If something unusual happens I'll refer the problem to the head nurse. Occasionally we develop our own methods for handling certain kinds of problems.

"I'm in charge of making sure the records are in order. That includes the physical and the history, which is a required part of the record. The physicians are supposed to do it within the first day after admission. A lot of them do it just before the patient is discharged and the record sent back to medical records. What can I say?" she shrugs.

"Taking care of messages is a big part of the job. A doctor will call up and say, 'Get so and so and tell them this.' I always hope and pray that I get the right message to the right person. After a while the people learn to trust you and you get a lot more messages.

"The desk clerks have a meeting each month with the director of nursing. We try to iron out problems that we have in common. For example, we have a lot of problems with the admissions department about emergency cases. We get them up on the floor and sometimes it's hours before we get plate—that's the blue plastic identification card we use. It is hard to get all the tests and stuff ordered without it. It's really infuriating. We have to fill out some of the forms by hand which isn't a very good idea. You'd think that emergencies would have priority in terms of producing cards for them, but I guess the admissions office doesn't see it that way. Things get better for a while after we make a fuss about it but then they slack off again."

Mary Ann pulls one of the blue plastic cards from the file. One of the doctors has returned a chart to the desk. He chats about the baseball game that he went to last night.

"Why is it this is such a city of losers?" he says. Several nurses gather around the desk. One is getting names for the hospital blood drive.

"How about you, Dr. Hall?" she says.

"Naw, I've got syphilis," he says.

"Aw, come on, we'll take foreign blood," another pipes in.

"Well, you see, I got hepatitis while I was in Spain a long time ago," he says, not joking this time. The nurse corners an orderly and starts twisting his arm.

"OK, I'll give in my department," the orderly says.

"But let me sign you up right now," the nurse persists. The doctor, who has been standing at the desk, finishes writing in the chart. "Take care," he says, leaving.

Mary Ann takes the chart and pulls the blue plastic ID card from the rack on the wall. She stamps several forms and fills them out—orders for lab tests—and then calls the dietary department. "Mr. Jones, on 4B, change his diet to a soft bland one for lunch . . . OK, fine."

"The night shift of nurses takes care of the diet orders for the day, but I have to check them because sometimes the physicians will change them after visiting the patients in the morning. There are times when people keep getting a pre-test liquid diet after the test is over. I try to track these things down and get the orders changed."

"Do you have the test results for Mrs. Sherwin?" asks a doctor. He has a yellow sports coat, greying hair, and a pleasant face. He drums his fingers on the counter.

"No, not yet. You want me to call and check?" Mary Ann asks.

The doctor nods.

After several minutes on hold, Mary Ann gets the lab and fills out a verbal lab report for the physician. The physician, however, has disappeared.

"It's frustrating at times. We get caught in the middle. The physicians want instant service and we have to try to get it from the lab. Sometimes it doesn't work quite that well." Mary Ann shrugs. "We're beginning to try out a primary nursing idea on the floors. In that case there wouldn't be a head nurse. Each nurse would be responsible for the complete care of five or six patients. The desk clerk would work for all of them. As it is now, the head nurse pretty much determines what the desk clerk's responsibilities are. Some of the desk clerks don't do as many things as I do. It depends."

Mary Ann calls the intensive care unit. "Hi, some of the lab reports on Mr. Jernegan were sent up here. Shall I send them up? OK . . . Hey, Sally," Mary Ann calls to a passing nurse. "Are you going up to the ICU?"

"Well, I wasn't planning to, but I'll drop them by on my way to lunch."

"Thanks . . . OK, they're on their way up."

The lunch trays have arrived and all the doctors have left. There is a lull in the activity around the nursing station. Mary Ann starts recording the afternoon blood pressure, temperature and pulse readings into the patient charts. The phone rings.

"No, Tillie doesn't work here. She's a patient. OK, I'll see she gets the message." Mary Ann hangs up. "Nancy, would you tell Tillie that her friend won't be coming in this afternoon. She has a virus."

The nurse who has just come out of the room opposite the nursing station nods.

As she sorts through the patient records, updating the blood pressure, temperature and pulse readings, a slip in one catches her attention. She dials the radiology department.

"Hi. We need to schedule a BE for Mrs. Harris. Saturday morning? OK, fine."

Several candy stripers walk past the station with a large vase of flowers.

"Hey, that's cute. Who is it for?" Mary Ann says.

The candy stripers point to a room down the corridor and Mary Ann nods approval.

An orderly arrives with a man in a wheelchair.

"I guess we won't make the trip until around 3:00," the orderly says.

"OK, I'll make sure Mr. Norris gets a lunch sent up," Mary Ann says. She dials the dietary department. "We send patients over to get bone scans at another hospital. The routine tests we do here. The CAT scans, which are three-dimensional X rays, are done over at the teaching hospital."

A few minutes later, a woman, the director of transportation, arrives on the floor.

"First they tell us one thing, then another," she grumbles. She gets Mr. Norris from his room. "Come on, Mr. Norris, looks like we're going now after all." She wheels him down the corridor. Mary Ann waves good-bye. Mr. Norris, looking confused, meekly returns the gesture.

Several doctors arrive at the nursing station.

"Hey, I was supposed to get a stat [lab test that is needed immediately] on Miller," one doctor says.

"Miller? He plays for the Reds," the other doctor says, looking up from a chart.

"Not our Miller," Mary Ann laughs. "They were confused about what you wanted. I got it straightened out."

The phone rings.

"Desk Clerk, 4B. No, she's gone up to the ICU."

At about two o'clock the activity on the floor slows down. Most of the physicians take Wednesday afternoons off. They come in early to see their patients. The filling out and dispatching of order forms slows down. The phone stops ringing. Several nurses sit at the desk chatting. The floor is quiet. Mary Ann can relax a little.

"It's been a really good experience here. I always wanted to be a nurse, but I was scared of the whole idea. Now I've had a chance to see it and become familiar with it all. Next fall I'm going to get into a practical nurse program."

At four o'clock the toilet at the end of the corridor overflows. Mary Ann calls maintenance.

"Look, I don't care if it is four-fifteen, George. You get up here and fix it... OK, forget about your ride. I'll drop you off. Come on, be a sport," Mary Ann smiles.

"After a while you get to know the people in the different departments. You know them as friends and you know which ones you can count on. Sometimes I ask specifically for a person I know I can work with and will get what I need. I can count on George."

At four-thirty Mary Ann is sorting through records and putting them in order. She throws out the verbal lab reports and puts the written ones into the patient records. She then finishes updating the drug and patient card files on the counter.

"Some people will just leave at four-thirty no matter what. I have to make sure that everything is in order. I'm just that way."

George comes out of the bathroom and signals his success by flashing a victory sign.

"Come on, Mary Ann. I play softball tonight," he says.

She takes one last check around the station; everything is in order. She joins George who is already waiting by the elevator.

SUMMARY

DUTIES: *Ward clerks assume responsibility for coordinating activities on patient floors: scheduling diagnostic tests, ordering meals, drugs and equipment for patients, updating medical records and such. In some hospitals there are service unit managers instead of ward clerks. Service unit managers are given more extensive administrative responsibilities than ward clerks and often report directly to the administrator, rather than the nursing supervisor. Hospitals differ in the way they organize these administrative responsibilities.*

TRAINING: *Mostly on-the-job training. Some junior colleges have special programs for training individuals for these responsibilities. A familiarity with the language and operation of a nursing floor plus an ability to deal tactfully but effectively with people will make one a desirable candidate.*

SALARY: *$8,000–18,000 depending on responsibilities and experience.*

12

BOARDING HOME OPERATOR

"Sunshine and Jennifer, stay here! Come back! Oh well, there they go."

Ellen Brandon shrugs and walks back to the kitchen door of the yellow three-story corner house. The two mongrel dogs disappear behind the hedge at the other end of the shady residential street.

The kitchen is large and sunny. A pot of coffee is warming on a two-burner hotplate in the corner. There is an oversized refrigerator next to it. On the opposite wall, a large counter with a dishwasher, sink and stove takes up most of the space. A rectangular chopping block island occupies the center of the room.

Ellen is having a cup of coffee in the breakfast nook that adjoins the kitchen. She is a small woman with red hair, in her early forties. Ellen and her husband Bob run a boarding home for the elderly. They fill an urgent need in the system of care for the aging. They provide a place for those who can't quite make it on their own, whose families cannot take them in, but who are too alert and healthy for a nursing home. Ellen and Bob run a house that is a real home for the boarders.

"It's funny how we got involved in this. Neither Bob nor I have any training in this area. I've gotten jobs on and off while the kids were growing up. I've always wavered between a full-time job and staying home all the time. I worked for a while, then stayed home, then went back and finished college. I taught for a while at a private school, then decided to take a year off. As usual, I got bored with staying home by the time Christmas came. I started working part-time for my uncle who has a mail order business, but that didn't do much for me either. He had a lot of routine work to do and wanted me to work more and more. I decided, heck, if I'm going to work I might as well do something interesting. I filled out a job application at the county welfare board. I didn't think anything was going to come of it, but three months later I got a call for an interview. They had to get a survey done for the federal government in three months, and they needed three extra people to finish it. It was interesting going around and talking to different people. After the survey was over they put me in the food stamp program and I interviewed people to determine whether they were eligible for food stamps. I enjoyed it."

The phone rings.

"Hi," Ellen answers. "How are you doing?... Gosh, I don't know whether anybody will like them, but we usually have a couple of vegetables at supper so we'll give it a try." She smiles and hangs up.

"That was a friend. His folks have a farm. He has an extra crate of mustard greens and wanted to know if we could use them. People are always calling us up and helping us out with things. Most of our friends know all of our boarders and make it a point to do something for them or pay them some attention when they come over. Sometimes they take them shopping or bring them something special.

"Anyway, working in the food stamp program got me interested in social service. I filled out an application to be a social service worker there at the welfare board. An opening came up several months later. They wanted someone to work helping people in the boarding homes. I didn't have the slightest idea what I was supposed to do or even what boarding homes were, but then I don't think anybody at the welfare board did either. We sort of made up the job as we went along. I started visiting the homes. The largest one is George Benson's. He used to run a chicken farm. But when the new airport was finished, the chickens couldn't handle the noise and the fumes and stopped laying. I guess he started out by taking in three patients from the state psychiatric hospital. There is an arrangement for farming them out that way. He began to realize there was more money in it than in eggs. So he started converting the chicken houses into rooms for boarders. He's grown tremendously since then. He's even hired a manager to run the show. He's now taking care of about 170 boarders.

"Physically, it's not quite as bad as it sounds, but they don't seem to really care about their people. It's an institution and not a home. At the beginning of each month they hand some of their boarders their Social Security checks face down to endorse. A lot of them are afraid to turn it over and see how much money they're really getting. That, to me, is the ultimate indignity, not to have control over your own money. Also, none of the boarders there are allowed to nap during the day. They figure that if they don't lie down they can shove them to bed early and they'll be easier to manage. All that kind of stuff makes me very angry. I mean, for a lot of these people the only thing they have left that makes them human is to be able to make choices for themselves. They are physically frail, a lot of them have no living relatives, or at least no living ones that care about them. If they can't make simple choices for themselves, what's left?"

A motorcycle rumbles into the driveway. Ellen's oldest son saunters into the kitchen and grabs a cup of coffee. He is a husky twenty-year-old and he's beaming.

"I passed the Taxi Driver's exam, mom," he says. He talks about the best ways to make money driving a cab. "A young woman was murdered last week downtown and now everybody's afraid of walking or taking the buses after dark. A lot more business for the cab drivers." He then goes back outside to tinker with the motorcycle.

Ellen smiles. "All three of our children are still living with us. They've all graduated from high school and now are trying out college and various jobs. Part of it is that apartments are really expensive. I guess, though, that the major thing that keeps us together is that Bob and I are so unflappable. Judy came in one night a few weeks ago and announced that she was going to move in with a guy. Bob and I looked at each other, shrugged, and started discussing what furniture she could have. She was furious. I'm sure she just wanted to get a rise out of us. Judy lives with us on the first floor, and the two boys have taken over the third floor of the house. All the boarders live on the second floor. The kids help out by moving furniture for the boarders and fixing the lamps and stuff. In turn, the boarders act like foster grandparents and really stick up for them. The boys had a spontaneous graduation party here a while back. Things got loud and noisy. I was worried that the boarders would be annoyed by it. When I asked them about it the next day they said the boys really deserved to have a good time and for me not to interfere.

"Working with many of the boarding homes for the welfare board was a real challenge. I did what I could for the boarders in the homes. I helped them to get financial or medical assistance. I got volunteers to come into the homes to do things with the people that lived there.

"One of the homes I tried to work with was this one. The people in it obviously needed some help, and the home itself was in pretty bad shape physically. But the lady who ran it didn't want to have anything to do with us. A while later I noticed a For Sale sign outside of it. The wheels began to turn in my head. Bob and I have never been very good with money, but since I was working we had been able to save a little. We were looking for a way to save it so we wouldn't be tempted to spend it, some income property or something. I had dragged the whole family out as volunteers in other homes, so they knew what it was all about.

"We're pretty impulsive about things. The next day we put $2,000 down on the house. It was only then that I started to worry about it. What if we couldn't sell our old house? We wouldn't have enough money to make up the difference between the selling price and the mortgage. I was having trouble sleeping. Bob said, 'So what? So we lose $2,000. Go to sleep.' He's always like that.

"It was pretty wild for the first six months. Nobody minded sharing their home with boarders though. Both the kids and Bob are pretty relaxed and low-keyed about things so I didn't have any worries about that. Besides, they had all enjoyed the volunteer work in the other homes.

"We've always had kids tramping through, staying for weekends, and friends dropping by. We're not really used to privacy and we like having people around. The house, though, was in horrible condition. For a while we were all working from six in the morning till midnight fixing things up. Now it's all pretty much under control and we've slowed down on the repair work.

"Bob and I talked quite a bit about how we wanted to run things. I wanted things to be open, to give the people as much independence and control over their lives as possible. If you don't have some independence and control over your life you can lose the desire to live. Independence is precious."

"Excuse me, Ellen, time to start getting things ready for lunch." A frail voice with an Irish lilt floats in from the dining room. A tiny woman with balding red hair enters the room hesitantly. Her thick glasses make her eyes appear twice their normal size.

"Oh, hi, Mary," Ellen says. "Yeah, I guess it's time I started pulling things together. No one would believe how unorganized and spur of the moment I am about the meals around here."

Ellen pulls some hamburger rolls out of the freezer and sticks them in the oven. She then cuts up some chicken and starts preparing a salad.

Mary collects some silverware and plates and carries them into the dining room.

"Hey, when's lunch going to be ready, Mary? This man is hungry," says a man sitting stiffly on a stuffed chair in the living room. He has one glass eye and a cane.

"Oh, be quiet and behave yourself, George. You're such a pest," says an overweight woman in a bathrobe, as she walks down the stairs. She smiles at George. Her face is warm and youthful. She starts to help Mary set the table. A larger man smiles from the other stuffed chair in the living room but continues staring at the ceiling, not moving.

Ellen finishes preparing the salad and gives it to Mary.

"OK, time to eat, everybody, come on," Mary says.

The rocking stops on the front porch and a somewhat younger man enters the front door. A heavyset woman from upstairs joins the group. They begin to eat. No one talks. The room appears dark in comparison to the kitchen.

Ellen returns to her seat in the breakfast nook with a sandwich of her own and another cup of coffee.

"We pretty much let the boarders run the show. We have our own living area on the first floor and they have theirs. I'm not allowed to go upstairs to the second floor where they have their rooms. Mary doesn't let me up there. They chase me out if I try to go up and help out with the cleaning. The only time I can is when the curtains need to be cleaned or when there are some major repairs. When Mary gets sick the others take over. Anna takes care of cleaning the bathroom. I prepare the meals and plan the shopping. Mary organizes the others. We stay out of things. We respect their privacy and they respect ours. I try never to make decisions for them, and I let them take responsibility for themselves.

"Ron, for example, is an alcoholic. I found out from the others that he was sneaking off downtown to see some of his old drinking buddies. When I gave him the thirty-dollar difference between his social security check and the board, I talked to him about it. I told him that it was his choice to do something about it, and although he wasn't disrupting things in the house, it wasn't good for him. I asked him whether he knew the number for AA. He said he did. So I let it go. He still went on drinking. But he always felt like he should come in and apologize to me. One time he did so right in the middle of a bridge game with some of my friends. It kind of startled them. I told him he didn't need to apologize to me, he hadn't bothered anyone with it, but he should decide to do something about it. He's let up quite a bit since then.

"We didn't have any trouble getting boarders for the house. Some of them, like Mary, were already here. We ran an ad for a while and got lots of calls. A lot of children are desperate to find a decent place for their parents to live. I don't blame them for not taking them in themselves. If my mother came here to live, I'd go out the window. With other peoples' parents, you don't get caught up in the past relationship and they can't push you around."

The phone rings.

"Hello . . . Yeah? What's the problem? No, we don't have any space now, but I can put you on the waiting list. What's the problem? . . . If you want I'll put you on the waiting list and call you if I get an opening." Ellen hangs up. "The woman has a sister working for Goodwill. Probably retarded or maybe an epileptic who was institutionalized.

"We have a long waiting list now. We don't advertise anymore. We get referrals from the nursing homes and from the welfare office. Sometimes physicians will refer people to us, old people who live in an unsafe neighborhood and aren't eating properly.

"We usually have eleven boarders here. One just left. It was a very sad situation. She had a lot of fears, but the major one was a fear of going to the hospital. She was nice to have around, active physically. She cleaned the bathroom, collected the trash and did sewing. She started having rectal bleeding. She didn't want me to know, but she told several of the women upstairs and swore them to secrecy. Of course they came right down and told me about it. My policy is not to interfere. I don't want them to clam up and not talk to me. I felt it had to be her decision to go to the doctor.

Eventually she talked to me about it and finally agreed to go see her old physician who only has office hours on Thursday. She must be one of his last patients. He told her to go into the hospital for tests. She was very fearful but put on a brave front. She packed a bag and told everybody she would be back in a couple of days. A different hospital had a fire and some of the patients were moved into the hospital where she was staying. She got confused and was convinced that her hospital was on fire. She got out of bed and started trying to get the other patients out of the hospital.

"They put her in a restraining jacket in an isolated room. Then she really flipped out. She was convinced that gangsters were after her. I suggested that they bring her back here to a place she was familiar with and maybe she would settle down. She was supposed to take tranquilizers, but she didn't. Things didn't work out. She wouldn't eat anything because she thought it was poisoned. She was convinced that gas was being piped in her room, and she threatened to jump out of a window if her son didn't come and get her. They have her heavily sedated and restrained in a nursing home now. Really sad. I kept hoping that she would come out of it.

"One of our other boarders had the same thing happen to him when he was sent to a hospital for an operation, and he snapped out of it. He got confused and wanted to leave. They strapped him down in a treatment room with a short nightgown. He was exposed and had nothing on his legs. When I got there he couldn't say a complete sentence. I talked to his physician about him and told him he shouldn't be in a room by himself. They put him in a room with another man and he pretty much came out of it. I can't see how anyone could stay sane in that situation."

Lunch is finished in the dining room. Mary comes into the kitchen and starts cleaning the counters. Anna, the heavyset woman, brings in the dishes. The others leave the table and disappear into other parts of the house.

"When we started out, I had lots of plans for activities for the boarders, but it hasn't worked out that way. They like their peace and quiet. They're not interested in getting involved in a lot of things. We don't have much in the way of planned activities, but a lot of things happen. It's haphazard, but I'm kind of that way so I don't mind. Everybody has her or his own routine. They are all different. Each has a different story to tell about her or his life, and different problems.

"Mary runs the house. I almost feel like an invader in her home. When I first came I felt guilty about not doing anything. The previous owner never did anything and Mary managed. Mary grew up in Ireland and came here as a teenager. Apparently she was a pretty gay liver, loved to dance and was always going out to nightclubs and bars with her friends. She had to quit her job in a canning factory because of a skin allergy. Now she has cataracts and is afraid to go out; she doesn't have any confidence. But she's still very alert.

"George is crippled and has to walk with a cane. He's blind in one eye. He can't read or write, and I don't think he can even tell time, but he's kind of memorized the television schedule so he has a rough idea of what time it is. He takes care of the fish for me now. He's very proud of that. He refers to them as 'his' fish. When I took him to the Social Security office for his interview he referred to me as his 'Mother.' He's a great kidder. When he first moved in he was very depressed because he was losing his sight. He was a diabetic. I persuaded his niece to send him to an eye doctor. He had cataracts. Even though he was eighty-three they operated on him. Everybody had just assumed they wouldn't. He made a fantastic recovery and now he is a different person. He does have a little trouble getting around. One of the boys saw him taking a leak off the front porch. I didn't say anything, though, cause I figured as soon as the downstairs bathroom was finished it wouldn't be a problem. I figure most things will resolve themselves if you don't get too upset about them. He watches TV in the evenings and usually goes to sleep about eight or eight-thirty unless there is a movie special. He was a dishwasher all his life, worked hard, lived in rooming houses."

Ellen pauses to check over her shopping list. It is a long one. She checks the refrigerator and adds milk and eggs to the list.

"We serve wine on Sundays to everybody, and on special occasions we have cocktails. It was kind of sticky at first because Ron is an alcoholic. But, I took my usual attitude that it was up to him, and he never drank a drop with us. He still sneaks some on the side. He has emphysema too. He would go out on the coldest mornings to get a cigarette. I caught him smoking on a really cold day on the porch. It was one of the few times I really flipped out. 'I can't believe you want to kill yourself,' I screamed at him. He got more secretive about it after that. He'd go smoke in the bathroom and the others would scold him. They're pretty good about looking after each other. He's in the hospital now. Reminds me, his seventy-eighth birthday is next week. I've got to take a present to him.

"Alice was a problem at first. She was on a ton of tranquilizers. I don't think she was ever very organized. She was very sloppy and would curse at her roommates. I mean, I don't care if she curses. But it upsets the others. I finally took her aside and told her that the reason I had this place was so people wouldn't have to take any crap from anybody. If you're angry come down and yell at me, don't bother your roommates. Anna was her roommate so I talked about the situation with her too. She didn't like Anna lying down on her bed after breakfast. You see she had been in George Benson's boarding home before she came here and they didn't allow anybody to lie down. So Alice would yell and scream at her. She was so programmed; she couldn't lie down herself. She didn't want anybody else to do it either. We've pretty much worked things out now, though.

"Anna is sweet, even-tempered and good-humored. She makes an effort. A few weeks ago George was crying because his niece was moving to Florida. She reached out to him and tried to cheer him up. Now they have a special thing going between them.

"The county welfare board sends a social worker out here to visit each week. She's been really helpful and has taken over a lot of things I used to do for the people. We had a big problem with Mary that the social worker helped out with. It seems that the woman who used to run the house would intercept the mail and cash her social security checks. Mary's brother found out about it. They didn't prosecute, but they made Mary sign something giving power of attorney to the brother's lawyer. They gave her five dollars a month spending money and they would sometimes drop off clothing for her from rummage sales. I guess they seemed to think they were doing her a favor by keeping her money. I couldn't deal with them because, of course, the brother and the lawyer were distrustful of me. I got the social worker to help. I was a little afraid Mary would give it all away, because that's the way she is. But then I thought it through and, after all, it is her money and she should be able to do with it what she wants to do.

"The social worker finally got the legal department at the welfare office to send a letter to the lawyer and it's all been straightened out now. She still doesn't get her check in her own name. The lady at the Social Security office was really snotty about it. Seems she had to get a doctor to certify that she could receive it. I asked how come if she signed it over voluntarily why couldn't she voluntarily get it back. She really didn't have an answer. Anyway, the doctor was more than happy to complete the required form. He wants us to go after *all* the money her brother was withholding. I suggested to Mary that she open a savings account. She is worried about having money for her burial, so she started one. She's really pleased about it. She can walk the three blocks down to the bank and deposit her own money. She then announced that she was now going to pay seventy dollars a week instead of sixty. It's ridiculous, I wanted to pay *her* but she was insulted and refused. I have a hard time giving her anything. She's a very proud, independent lady. We had a battle over the raising of the rent. 'But Mary, everybody in this whole country is complaining about the landlord raising the rent and you want to pay more,' I'd tell her. I thought maybe Bob could deal with her better, but she was just as stubborn with him. We've finally had to give in on it.

"Mary's real concern was with Elizabeth. Elizabeth rubbed it in that she had a private room and 'put on airs.' Mary wanted to show her she was just as good. It was really awful what happened to Elizabeth though. She's eighty-three and an old maid. She had worked for RCA, had a nice pension, and lived in what used to be a good neighborhood until it started to get run down. She was an easy target. The third day of the month was social security check day and she was robbed three times. They'd hold a knife to her throat in bed and force her to tell them where the money was. It got to the point where she was afraid to sleep in bed and would sleep downstairs in her rocking chair. There was somebody down the street who was worse off than she but made sure she got a meal every day. But Elizabeth got sick. A neighbor found her passed out on the floor with pneumonia. She was hospitalized, spent some time in a nursing home and then came to us.

"She brought a lot of her own furniture with her. Her room is filled with her old stuff and we have a lot stored in the basement. We had a real problem with her at first. She's hard of hearing and would fall asleep in her rocking chair with the TV blaring away in front of her. When I'd go in and try to wake her up she'd fly off the seat screaming, thinking somebody had come back to rob her at knife point. The same thing started happening in the bathroom. She'd fall asleep on the toilet. When some of the others would try to wake her up, she'd be really scared by it. But, she's gradually calmed down. She's not as fearful as she was at first.

"Then there's Frank, he's another favorite of mine. He's blind, gets along well with everybody. He has a wonderful friend he met in town at a Horn and Hardart automat. His name is Jimmy. They struck up a conversation and they've been close friends since then. Jimmy is a very gregarious guy with a young family. He storms through here, gives Tony a Cuban cigar and kids around with everybody. Frank used to visit Jimmy's family regularly and go on special vacation outings. Last Christmas, he came back a little shell-shocked. Three young children are probably hard to take in large doses if you're not used to them. This Christmas he told Jimmy he had a cold and stayed with us. He didn't really, but I guess he didn't want to hurt Jimmy's feelings. He calls this place the Mansion and I think he feels pretty much at home here. I'd really like to have him more active, but he doesn't really want anything to do. Most of the day he spends just listening to the radio. George invites him to watch the Lawrence Welk show with him. Everybody watches the Lawrence Welk show here except, of course, Frank, who can't see anything, but that doesn't matter.

"Tony is different from the others. He's a Cuban refugee. He was a well-to-do wholesale grocery businessman in Havana before the revolution. He had a seashore home, maids and all that. They took everything away from him when he left. Even took his wife's gold wedding band off as they were getting in the plane to fly to Miami. That wedding band was more important than all the rest to Tony. He gets furious when he thinks about it. He's a super United States patriot now, although he hasn't gotten his citizenship yet. He has had a very hard time with the language. He still can't speak English well. He wasn't able to get any decent work in the States, partly because of the language problem. He has had three nervous breakdowns since coming to the States.

"Tony has a very macho outlook on things. Not being able to support his family put a tremendous strain on him. After the last breakdown, the psychiatrist recommended that he not go back to his family and he came to live with us. He's just sixty and physically not in bad shape. He takes care of the yard work. I've also made him responsible for the garage key. If I give it to him, he always knows where it is. I know a little Spanish, so I am able to talk to him. He's OK with the written stuff but he can't communicate with others. I tried to get him involved in a night class in English for foreigners but it was too hard for him and he got discouraged. I usually take him with me when I go grocery shopping. He knows a lot about the grocery business and is very helpful.

"I give the boarders a lot of freedom but I guess they're still afraid and can't be completely free with me. I have asked people to leave. There was one woman who kept smoking in bed. Nobody is allowed to smoke upstairs. She kept falling asleep smoking and setting fires. She had spent the first sixty years of her life at a school for the retarded, although I really doubt whether she was retarded. She went to a lot of different places after she left here.

"We're not a licensed boarding home yet, and I'm not sure we want to be. We'd get another $100 a month from welfare if we were, though. Right now we only get $200 a month from the welfare office. Half of our people, however, pay their own way, either out of Social Security or their own pensions. Elizabeth pays $343.90 a month for her private room. Don't ask me how we figured out that.

"I don't know whether we're psychologically ready for licensing yet. The inspector came by to look at the home and was very encouraging. She said a lot of the requirements could be waived temporarily. I know we can't have a laundry in the back bathroom, since it's connected to a food preparation area. The main thing is, though, that we couldn't have any of the boarders work. We'd have to pay them at least minimum wage. I've tried to pay Mary but she won't take it. I don't know what we'd do. You can measure how fast they do the work and adjust their pay that way, but it would be an awful amount of paperwork and red tape and I'm just not sure we want to bother with it.

"We just about broke even on the operation last year, but there were an awful lot of costly repairs. Next year, after we take out all the cost, we should make eight or nine thousand dollars. Not much, but then this really isn't a business and we're not just doing it for the money."

Ellen picks up her shopping list and heads for the back door.

"So long, everybody, I'll see you at supper time," she says, not looking back.

George nods and waves from his chair in the living room. None of the others is downstairs. The house is quiet.

SUMMARY

DUTIES: *A boarding home operator provides a sheltered home for the elderly and disabled. S/he is responsible for providing meals to the boarders, supplying laundry and housekeeping services and assisting boarders in obtaining medical and social welfare services.*

TRAINING: *There are no formal educational requirements. Some states and local health or welfare departments require that the operators be licensed. Applicants for such licenses must be of "good character" and demonstrate sufficient competence to undertake such an effort. In addition, most states and local health or welfare departments license the facilities themselves. Check with these agencies about the requirements in your area.*

SALARY: *$6,000–20,000, depending on the size and licensure status of the home.*

13

HOSPITAL ADMINISTRATOR

Jim Walsh swings the car onto a side street and then into the alley behind the old hospital. At six-thirty in the morning, all the parking spaces are vacant. He pulls into one, turns off the car lights, climbs out and stretches. Rowhouses line the opposite side of the street. Metal has been tacked over some of the windows, sealing out sunlight and neighborhood intruders. The car of an early morning commuter rustles the newspapers in the gutter, as Jim walks toward the entrance of the old hospital where the administrative offices are located. The white cement buildings of the medical center now engulf the older brick building. Jim exchanges nods with the guard at the door and passes into the cool, quiet, carpeted wood-paneled interior. Oil paintings of former faculty members of the medical school line the hall adjacent to his office.

He grabs a stack of mail and memorandums off his secretary's desk, passes into his own office and sinks down in the captain's chair next to his antique roll top desk. There are notes from department heads making special appeals for equipment, some written patient complaints and a bid by a consulting firm for putting a new concrete floor in the older building. He makes notes on what is to be done on each and who is to handle it. There is also a large assortment of junk mail that needs to be emptied into the wastepaper basket. "I come in early to keep this stuff from piling up. It's usually the only time I can go through these things." He wanders back into the secretary's office to make some instant coffee.

At eight, Donna Wilson, the administrative secretary, comes in with the morning mail and he passes on these notes to her. "Hi, Donna. Ed Paley should take a look at this letter. There's a lot more involved in it, I think." He hands her all of the material he's gone through. Donna nods.

Jim sips his second cup of coffee and continues to review the stack of correspondence and journals on his desk.

"Like a lot of people, I sort of fell into doing this kind of work. I was working on a doctorate in history at Columbia and I got a job as an elevator operator at Columbia Presbyterian Hospital. Then I got a job in central supply. You know, where all the sheets and linen and a lot of equipment used on the nursing floors are kept. It was a pretty routine kind of job, but I got to be in contact with all parts of the hospital. I got seduced by it all. It was intricate, complex, sometimes full of drama. History studies began to seem pretty dry by comparison. Eventually, I went and got a degree in Hospital Administration. I don't regret it, history is still a hobby for me. But you know, it's not that different, universities and hospitals are pretty much the same in a lot of ways."

"A while back, I got really depressed about it all. In this job you never get a pat on the back. People are always angry with you. I talked to somebody about it. He said, 'Look, Jim, you're the inkblot of the institution. Whatever people feel about the hospital is reflected in how they deal with you. It really is not you, it is the hospital they're reacting to. Also, you've got to remember you're the focus of discontent. If medical staff members get into a fight over something they blame it on you. It's easier than dealing with the problem themselves.'

"That's the way it is and it's important to keep it in mind. It's just like in the rest of the university down the street. The faculty is always blaming the administration for screwing up the university. The basic conflict between an administrator and the medical staff is that I'm the provider and they're the consumer. They want the very best, but I'm the one who's held accountable for having the money to pay for it. The more the medical staff has, the more status they get. There's no incentive for them to do with less. It's the same thing in all the hospital departments, everybody feels that the more people they supervise, the more important they are and the more status they have. Everybody wants an administrative assistant.

"Then there's the whole problem of dividing up space in the hospital. There is a lot of space in the building that isn't really used well, but it's like pulling teeth to get one group to give it up. My job is to take it away from the haves and give it to the have nots. No matter what you do you lose. The have nots never feel you have given them enough and the haves feel personally slighted. They feel you don't appreciate what they're doing and think you don't have any respect for them, but what can you do?" He shrugs. "Physicians, just like most other professional groups, resent being told what to do. They resent boundaries and administrators are paid to take the flack.

"As an institution, we need goals and objectives, but it's really hard to get agreement. There's a lot of distrust between different groups in a hospital this size. Hospitals like this are full of conflicts. The nurses and the medical staff are always squabbling over who should do what. Nurses are now trained to do a lot more than they used to and they want to use their skills, but physicians often feel threatened. Then, of course, everybody wants to get rid of the more disagreeable tasks and do the more exotic, fancy stuff. For example, aides do the enemas instead of the nurses. It's not a very pleasant thing to do, but it may not be the right thing to delegate to less trained people because you can really harm somebody if you don't know exactly what you're doing. But of course, they're no different than everybody else. The surgeons have surgical technicians doing most of the routine accident stuff in the emergency rooms and even the social workers have social work technicians to handle the more routine paper processing. Everybody wants to pass on the less desirable work to somebody else.

"It's funny, there aren't many conflicts between the nursing aides and the registered nurses. They usually don't talk to each other. The aides are just assigned a task, like taking temperatures, and that's it. They're kind of invisible people as far as the nursing staff is concerned. Nurses don't feel comfortable giving orders to them or talking to them. Maybe it's because most of the aides are black and the nurses white, but I've seen the same thing in other settings when this really wasn't the case. At any rate, it's not surprising that the aides were the first to be unionized.

"There are other black and white differences. There seem to be black and white jobs in the hospital. Housekeeping and the telephone room are black jobs; engineering and maintenance is a white job. It's really rough for people who cross the line from either side. Black employees in the maintenance department usually don't last and it's really rough the other way too. We put a white woman into the telephone room a few months ago and she had a really tough time. The people did not like her 'taking away a job from a black.' I wish that the black physicians on our staff were a little more visible, not stuck away in the labs. It's been really slow going opening things up.

"Physicians contribute to the number of conflicts. The radiologists and the orthopedic surgeons are always at each others' throats and somehow there always seems to be a lot of conflict between the internal medicine faculty and the dietary department.

"The surgical technicians have created a lot of problems too. For a long time they were only responsible to the medical staff in a nebulous kind of way. It was kind of like when I started work in the hospitals in the 50s. MDs used to bring their own obstetrical nurses or surgical nurses with them when they came to a hospital. They wanted people who were used to the way they worked. Of course when hospitals lost their charitable immunity and could be sued, hospitals started to get concerned, set up standards and insisted on using only their own staff in the delivery and surgical suites.

"It was the same sort of thing here. There was a lot of conflict with the nursing staff about what the surgical techs were doing. One of the first things I did when I became administrator here was to put the techs under the control of the nursing department. Of course that didn't make a lot of the surgical techs very happy. Six of them quit. They were trained in medical schools and had adopted a lot of the physicians' prejudices about nurses. Now the shoe's on the other foot and the surgical techs complain to one of the doctors about their treatment and then the doctor complains to the director of nurses and then sometimes we get involved. The whole situation, though, is still in a state of flux."

Donna buzzes him.

"Excuse me, it's eight-thirty and John and Bob are here to talk about the capital budgets."

"OK, I'll join them in the conference room in just a minute," Jim says.

"A teaching hospital is more complex than most community hospitals," he explains. "I'm what's called 'Mr. Outside.' I deal with the university, the medical school and any outside bodies that regulate us. John Lawton is the inside man. He handles the hospital departments and the day to day stuff within the hospital—housekeeping, dietary, laboratories, maintenance and so forth. Both of us spend a lot of time in meetings. People feel more comfortable about that kind of coordination, although I keep feeling we should be able to figure out a better way to do it."

Jim grabs several folders and walks to the small conference room on the other side of his secretary's office.

John Lawton and Bob Walker are poring over figures and reports that are spread on the table.

Bob Walker is the financial director for the hospital. He's heavy-set and pensive. He's been with the hospital more than fifteen years.

"You want to know what administrators do?" he says, "They spend a lot of time crying."

John Lawton appears more relaxed and quiet.

The meeting has to do with the capital budgets for the hospital. Capital budgets include money to renovate and refurbish old facilities, money to purchase new equipment and money to construct new facilities. There's not much to spread around. The hospital lost $2.5 million last year. Many of the clients are poor and can't afford to pay. Even if they are eligible for Medicaid, the state Medicaid program only covers a portion of what it costs the hospital to provide care. The three men look for ways out of the squeeze.

They talk about the advantages of leasing equipment instead of purchasing it, as has been done in the past. Leasing costs more in the long run, but if an organization is short on money, it's a way of freeing it for other projects and offsetting deficits. Blue Cross and Medicare give them money for capital depreciation in addition to the costs of providing patient care. Like many urban hospitals, they are dipping more and more into this money to help pay for rising operating costs. If the funds are used this way, there will be no money to build a new hospital when it is needed. But right now the hospital just wants to survive. They don't have the luxury of planning too far into the future.

They discuss the JCAH (Joint Commission on Accreditation of Hospitals) report. The Joint Commission certifies the adequacy of hospitals. The last inspection team recommended disaccreditation. That could mean that third party reimbursement sources, such as Medicare and Medicaid, might no longer pay for services provided in the hospital. The hospital needs the money that comes from those sources in order to operate. It is appealing the decision and trying to decide how to show the surveyors that the deficiencies have been corrected.

"How do we handle the nurse staffing issue?" Jim asks. "They were really vague. What kind of staffing ratio do you think would satisfy them?" The three of them mull this over for a while, along with the costs implied by additional staffing.

"Thank God we didn't sign the contract for putting in the new sprinkler system as that earlier team told us to do," John says. "This year's inspection team recommended concrete floors instead."

"The JCAH is under fire from consumer groups now. I guess it feels it has to show a good box score," Jim explains. "You know, they have to show how many hospitals they disaccredited this year. They've been criticized for being a bunch of 'foxes guarding a hen house.' Now they want to prove they're tough, but that's not really what that program was ever supposed to do. Now they go about nit-picking. The inspectors want to catch you at something so they can prove they're tough."

The discussion returns to the capital budget.

"We've got to zero in on a contract with an interior design firm. We need a firm that will develop the standards for design and color coding of floors and equipment and so forth. The remodeling we've done already may be wasted without it. We've got to have a plan put together fast."

"Interspace got the contract in Bowman, North Carolina," John says.

"Yeah, well, we'd all like to use a firm we've worked with before. But the main thing is that we've got to get going on this right away." Jim taps his hand on the table to emphasize his point.

"What about the private practice units. Do we have any control over what they purchase?"

"Yes, we're the landlord, but we'd have a hard time making it stick," Bob answers.

"Psychiatry is going ahead with its own purchasing of new furniture. We could tell them to go to hell," John says.

"Look, let's get on top of this, give these departments an approved list of things they can pick. We'll be better off if we give them some positive choices rather than just saying 'no.' "

"Let's try to give them some options."

"Bob, let's write some performance specifications for the medical equipment. It's unheard of and we'll need a professional advisory committee to help us," Jim continues, as he ticks off mental notes to the other two administrators.

"How about the Student and Personnel Health situation?" Jim asks. "Get hold of Norma, John, and see what we can do. We should figure out how we can work effectively with them."

"Well, Local 1199 was dissatisfied with the physician in the Personnel Health Service, but it hasn't been changed," Bob answers. "There was also a medical student who had a series of allergy shots and didn't realize it wasn't going to come out of his Blue Cross/Blue Shield. He tried to get the hospital to write off his bill. I told him no dice. I know the medical school gets something off the top from those BC/BS premiums. They've got a slush fund set up for just that kind of thing. I told him to go see the Dean."

"OK, let's get back on the JCAH stuff tomorrow. I've got to get down to campus for a meeting. Catch you for lunch, John."

"Yeah, OK," John says.

Ron Dexter, the new administrator with a systems analyst background, enters the office just as Jim is leaving.

"Hey Ron, take a look at this stuff. You notice it's the large medical centers in the city that are always running short. See what you can make out of it."

Ron grabs the tables and peers intently at the statistical summaries from all of the metropolitan hospitals.

"Sure, OK, I'll see what I can do . . ."

Jim heads for his car through the back door.

"I brought Ron on because I figured what we needed more than anything else was a good systems analyst. Somebody who could cut through all the concern about turf in this place. We've been talking about getting all of our blood from Red Cross rather than having our own program within the hospital. There are a lot of costs involved if we have to have a cross matching team, which is a group that tests blood compatibility before transfusions, and the equipment. It costs roughly $100,000 a year to operate. But, last week Red Cross ran out of blood. So, what do you do? We don't want to use the commercial blood banks, you know those inner city storefront operations. The blood from them costs more and there's always the danger of hepatitis. Maybe Ron can figure out the answer."

Jim drives the several miles that separate the medical school from the rest of the campus. He is heading for a committee meeting on the main campus.

"This commuting back and forth is a pain, but it's important to let them know that we exist up here. I asked to be on the administrative systems committee partly because I wanted to protect turf. Not so much in an administrative sense but just to make people aware of the impact on us of decisions that were made. For example, the university closed down for a couple of weeks after Christmas last year to save on fuel. But, of course, the hospital couldn't. What had they done about compensation of the employees and so forth? They hadn't thought about that.

"We're a different kind of operation. We have to make sure we mesh with the rest of the university. My other official title is Vice-President for Health Services. So, part of my job is to coordinate the activities of the medical center with the rest of the campus."

The university administration building is across the street from where Jim parks his car. He enters the building and takes the elevator to the top floor. The doors open up on wide carpeted corridors. The meeting is scheduled in the president's conference room. Five of the other university vice-presidents are present.

"You think our meetings are bad," one of the vice-presidents says, stuffing his pipe, "you should go to the Health System Agency meetings. It's like going to a Mad Hatter's tea party!"

The final member arrives and they get down to working on the agenda for the meeting. When the meeting is over, Jim stretches as the others leave the conference room.

"George, can I have a few seconds of your time?"

"Sure, give me a few minutes. I've got a phone call."

"I wonder whether in twenty years there will be another group sitting around that same table, wondering, just as we have been, how people running the place twenty years ago could have been so stupid," Jim says.

Jim walks down the wide corridor to the office of George Bronson, financial vice-president, who chaired the meeting.

George hangs up the phone and Jim enters his office. George leans back in the swivel chair behind his desk, hands behind his head. Jim paces in front of him.

"Look, I just want to alert you to what's happening at the student cafeteria up at the medical school campus. I told Bill up there that our hospital dietary department might make a bid to run it, but he didn't seem very interested. He's going to take the lowest bid from an outside firm without taking anything else into account. I'm not sure but I could make a good case for the hospital dietary department taking over the operation. For one thing, we could expand the service to more than just lunches. For another, there's a hell of a lot of space over there and we could possibly move the whole dietary department over there and free up some space within the hospital."

"OK, go ahead and develop the idea," George says. "It seems like a good one."

Jim leaves George Bronson's office and joins John Lawton at a restaurant near the hospital. They munch on tuna salad and crackers. The dark interior of the restaurant seems well removed from the hospital.

Instead of going back to the office after lunch, Jim makes the rounds of the hospital. He enters the elevator and gets off at the top floor.

"Making rounds is more symbolic than anything else. You're 'showing the flag.' Administrators are always accused of never getting off the first floor and seeing what happens on the patient floors. It's important that you show up on the floors, it's a way of acknowledging the importance of the work that goes on there."

He looks down the hallway past the nursing station.

"This part of the hospital was built in the 1950s and before they finished, it was out of date. People think that because it's newer than the old hospital, it's OK, but there just isn't enough space for all the equipment that is now used. There's no place to store it and it gets stacked up in the corridors. It's hard for the staff to work around."

He glances at the inhalation therapy equipment, a drug dispensing cart, some of the cleaning equipment tucked along the wall of the corridor and waves at a nurse at the desk. He opens the door to go down to the next level. The second fire door enclosing the stairwell is open.

"You see that door? That would be cited for a violation if a state inspector came through. We have signs saying that they must be closed at all times, but with all the people using the stairs, how do you control it? Anyway, how important is it really? The signs are there. The door could be easily closed in the event of a fire. Wouldn't it make more sense to concentrate on something like medication errors that have a much more direct effect on patients?"

"Here's the most difficult space problem," he says, opening the door to the intensive care unit.

It consists of two hospital rooms that have been converted by knocking out a wall. The beds are filled. Eight frail bodies crowded together, concealed from each other by IVs, respirators, cardiac monitors and a hovering nursing staff. There's little room for the staff to maneuver between the jumble of wires and tubes.

Jim winces and closes the door.

Father Jackson, the Catholic chaplain, bumps into him in the corridor of the older section of the hospital.

"Hi, what's been happening? Everything under control?" the priest asks. He is young, bearded, and has a mischievous look on his face.

Jim laughs. "The answer to the first question is, you know as much as me and to the second, no."

They both laugh. Jim heads back to the office.

Just outside, he meets Ed Paley, the person who handles the malpractice and liability problems within the hospital.

"Hi, Ed, did you have a chance to look at that letter?"

"Yeah. I think you're right about there being more to it. I'm going to dig out the record this afternoon and pull together the material on it."

"OK, good."

Jim returns to his office. Donna hands him the afternoon mail.

"Ed's our inhouse legal paraprofessional. I guess they call them 'risk managers' today. He started out in the maintenance department, but he probably knows more about malpractice law and hospital liability than most lawyers. We have paid out very little in malpractice and liability damages. Part of that is because we provide good care, but part of it's also because if there's a potential problem, Ed jumps in and heads it off early. You know, talking to the family and patient and so forth."

He checks over the mail. There's a letter from the Joint Commission. He dials John Lawton's number.

"Hi, John, just got a letter from the JCAH confirming the meeting on the 20th at two in the afternoon. They also enclosed a list of hotels. Oh, I guess it's about an hour and a half flight to Chicago. Yeah, we could probably get back in one day. Anyway, we have to figure who we're going to take. We also have to talk about strategy."

His phone conversation ended, Jim sighs and stretches back in his chair.

"These guys on the inspection teams have reams of material they have to sift through. They hunt for weaknesses. It's turned into an adversary process now. The JCAH inspectors tend to be pretty rigid in the way they interpret things. The central office staff of the JCAH is pretty sensible, much better than the staff of the state health department. Those guys have too limited a view of things," he sighs.

"A hospital administrator doesn't get narrowed down into a small specialized area the way bureaucrats do. It's one of the more satisfying things about this work—the variety. You have to know about liability and malpractice risks, health insurance reimbursement, the basics of running a large physical plant, the kind of relationship your hospital has to the community it serves and you have to be plugged into the local political arena."

Donna comes in and hands him some more mail.

"Thanks, I'll look it over tonight. I'm off to the University Board of Trustees meeting."

As a vice-president, Jim routinely attends these meetings to answer questions about the hospital. The hospital is under fire because of the $2.5 million deficit. Some of the trustees would like to get rid of the hospital so that the university, which is in increasingly bad financial shape itself, would not have to continue to bail out the hospital.

"What they don't understand is that some of the medical school salaries and equipment are paid for by the hospital. If the university cuts ties with the hospital, they'll probably lose $6 million instead of saving $2.5 million. Over the summer, we put together a document. We then went individually to each board member and tried to explain the problem. I hope that the message got through and that it won't be an issue today."

The board of trustees meeting is in a large amphitheater on the main campus. The twenty-two board members sit in the front row next to microphones. Jim, some of the other vice-presidents, faculty and student representatives sit in the back rows. At four-thirty the meeting is over and Jim heads for another meeting downtown.

"I've got meetings every night this week. Most of the time nothing is accomplished, but you have to protect the interest of the hospital and if you miss one, there's a chance you might have to deal with some nasty surprises. The meeting tonight, however, is different. It's a community leadership seminar. Several local groups sponsor it and they try to recruit people from different backgrounds in the city who have a chance of shaping things. There are representatives of the banks, law offices, government, large corporations, the news media and some hospital administrators like myself. It's very worthwhile. We have readings ahead of time and knowledgeable people come in and speak. It also helps to create some good communication between people in other areas of the city that you can call on later."

Jim swings back into the main thoroughfare and heads toward the center of the city. The traffic is light. The commuters are all heading in the opposite direction.

In the hospital, food trays are being delivered to the floors. Relatives of patients, some drained and tense, stand by the reception desk waiting to get visitor passes. The evening shift in the ICU has begun their crowded vigil. A bullet wound of a young man is being sewed up by a resident in the emergency room. The hospital continues to work.

SUMMARY

DUTIES: *The administrator is responsible for the overall operation of an acute-care hospital. In hospitals with more than a hundred beds there will usually be several assistant administrators responsible for the operation of certain departments within the hospital. Duties include: the financial management of the institution, the purchase of new equipment, the planning of new programs and facilities and the overall supervision of hospital departments such as the laboratory, pharmacy, medical records and so forth.*

TRAINING: *Most states do not have licensure requirements, but many hospitals now require a master's degree from an accredited program in hospital or health services administration. For more information, contact:*

> *Association of University Programs in Health Administration*
> *One Dupont Circle, Suite 132*
> *Washington, D.C. 20036*

SALARY: *$12,000–80,000 depending on responsibilities, and size and location of the hospital.*

RELATED OCCUPATIONS

NURSING HOME ADMINISTRATOR

DUTIES: *Responsible for the operation of a facility that provides 24-hour nursing care to chronically ill, mostly elderly patients. Since visits by physicians may be infrequent and there is little in the way of an organized medical staff, the nursing home administrator is usually far more directly involved in patient care than is an administrator in a hospital.*

TRAINING: *A number of states require nursing home administrators to be licensed. This may involve some educational requirements and an exam. Check with local health departments about the requirements. A background in either business administration or nursing is helpful. There are some undergraduate programs in health administration that specialize in training nursing home administrators. An increasing number of nursing home administrators are obtaining master's degrees in health administration. For information about both the undergraduate and graduate programs, write:*

*Association of University Programs in Health Administration
One Dupont Circle, Suite 132
Washington, D.C. 20036*

SALARY: *$10,000–50,000 depending on the size and location of the facility.*

PERSONNEL ADMINISTRATOR

DUTIES: *Provides assistance to the various departments in the hospital in dealing with their personnel needs. This includes analyzing the positions required by each department, assisting in the selection of job applicants and determining the wages that will be paid to different employees. They also are usually responsible for some of the orientation and training of new employees. In addition to an administrator, a personnel department often includes an employment manager, responsible for interviewing and screening job applicants, a job analyst who collects information on how to select and pay employees and someone responsible for the orientation and on-the-job training of employees.*

TRAINING: *Work experience in personnel administration, undergraduate or graduate training in personnel administration in a business school or a combination of the two.*

SALARY: *$12,000–25,000 depending on responsibilities.*

REGISTERED RECORDS ADMINISTRATOR

DUTIES: *Establishes and maintains a system of medical records that is accurate, complete and accessible. The administrator usually serves on the utilization review committee that determines whether physicians are using hospital beds appropriately; the medical audit committee that reviews the quality of care provided patients; and the medical records committee of the medical staff which assists the records administrator in obtaining timely and complete records on patients. In a large teaching hospital the administrator may be responsible for supervising fifty or more employees, such as technicians and assistants who process and retrieve records and perform the audits and special studies requested by the medical staff committees.*

TRAINING: *Registered records administrators have a four-year Bachelor of Science degree from an accredited program in medical records administration. The program includes courses in personnel administration, budgeting, computer information systems and biostatistics. They must pass a national exam given by the American Medical Record Association. Programs are jointly accredited by the American Medical Record Association and the Council on Medical Education of the American Medical Association. For more information, contact:*

> *American Medical Record Association*
> *875 North Michigan Avenue*
> *Chicago, Illinois 60611*

SALARY: *$12,000–30,000 depending on size of supervisory responsibilities and experience.*

ACCREDITED RECORD TECHNICIAN

DUTIES: *Serves as an administrator of a medical records department, a medical audit assistant or assists in carrying out the other responsibilities of a hospital record department. Also, may serve as records consultant to nursing homes.*

TRAINING: *High-school graduate or equivalent, some typing ability. The individual may take a two-year junior college Medical Records Technician program, accredited by the American Medical Record Association, or a correspondence course offered by the association. The association will assign a registered records administrator to serve as tutor and evaluator of the student's progress in the correspondence course. S/he must then pass the national exam of the Association to be accredited. For information about the correspondence and junior college programs, contact:*

>   *American Medical Record Association*
>   *875 North Michigan Avenue*
>   *Chicago, Illinois 60611*

SALARY: *$10,000–20,000 depending on administrative responsibilities and experience.*

FINANCIAL MANAGER

DUTIES: *Sometimes referred to as the controller, chief financial officer or business services manager, s/he acts as chief financial officer and supervisor to the business office of the hospital. S/he is responsible for both collecting money for the hospital from insurance companies, public agencies and patients, and for supplying the money to pay salaries and purchase equipment for the hospital. S/he establishes the procedures for keeping track of this flow of money.*

TRAINING: *An undergraduate background in accounting or business administration with a heavy emphasis on accounting. Individuals should have experience with accounting problems in health settings and with supervisory responsibilities. Specialized training programs in health-care financial management are now provided at several universities. Contact the Association of University Programs in Health Services Administration for information. Also, the Hospital Financial Management Association provides correspondence courses, annual institutes and certification for those working in this area. For more information, contact:*

Hospital Financial Management Association
660 N. Lake Shore Drive
Chicago, Illinois 60611

SALARY: *$20,000–60,000: good financial managers are in high demand.*

HEALTH PLANNER

DUTIES: *Estimates future needs of health services and plans how these needs can best be met. Works for the newly created Health Systems Agencies that are responsible for planning health services within a region or for hospitals or public agencies. Planners who work for health facilities plan the construction of new facilities and the development of new services and programs. Planners who work in Health Systems Agencies review the construction projects of local health facilities to determine whether they are needed and assist in developing coordinated programs to deal with community health problems.*

TRAINING: *Master's degree in health planning or health services administration, although individuals with a wide variety of backgrounds are currently working in this area. For more information, contact:*

American Association of Comprehensive Health Planning
801 North Fairfax Street
Alexandria, Virginia 22314

SALARY: *$12,000–50,000 depending on administrative responsibilities.*

HEALTH INSURANCE PLAN ADMINISTRATOR

DUTIES: *Responsible for assisting in the administration of a health insurance plan. Plans range from the multi-billion-dollar public insurance programs such as Medicare and Medicaid, the large billion-dollar regional Blue Cross plans and national commercial insurance plans to small independent plans run by local labor unions and employers. Some insurance programs just pay the bills sent to them by hospitals, physicians or those who subscribe to the insurance plan. Others, sometimes called "Health Maintenance Organiza-*

tions," are directly involved in providing services. In any event, administrators are responsible for paying some of the costs of health care of their subscribers, doing it efficiently, avoiding deficits and attempting to exert influence on the providers of those services so that their subscribers can get the most for their money. Large health insurance plans employ people with specialized expertise in actuarial science, computer and information science, accounting and finance. Increasingly, they also hire responsible individuals for investigating fraud and abuse of the insurance plan by the providers of services.

TRAINING: *Insurance plans require some people with highly specialized skills and some administrative generalists. Top administrative positions are usually filled through promotion from within.*

SALARY: *$25,000–80,000 depending on responsibilities.*

MEDICAL SECRETARY

DUTIES: *Responsible for most of the business functions in a physician's office and for coordinating patient-care activities. The medical secretary schedules appointments, handles incoming calls, maintains financial records for the practice and handles patient fee payments. S/he may also be involved in more direct patient-care activities such as weighing patients, preparing them for examination by the physician, providing patients with medications under the physician's orders and performing some routine diagnostic tests.*

TRAINING: *Requires basic secretarial skills including typing, shorthand, bookkeeping and a familiarity with business law. S/he must also be familiar with medical terminology, medical records systems and health insurance forms and procedures. Two-year junior college programs are available. For more information, contact:*

> National Registry of Medical Secretaries
> P.O. Box 360
> Newton Highlands, Mass. 02161

SALARY: *$6,000–16,000 depending on experience, location and responsibilities.*

LABOR ORGANIZER

DUTIES: *Assists in union drives to represent employees in collective bargaining negotiations with health facilities. May also participate in contract negotiations for union members and in handling job grievance problems for workers.*

TRAINING: *Many organizers are health workers who become organizers as a result of unionization efforts. As with most jobs within unions, training is largely on the job. Some have received special training in schools of industrial and labor relations. For further information, contact local unions of hospital and health-care employees.*

SALARY: *$8,000–18,000 depending on experience and responsibilities.*

protectors of health

No area in health care has gotten as much recent attention as prevention. Prevention, or at least certain preventive programs, have the biggest payoff in improving people's health. Most improvement in life expectancy in the last one hundred years can be attributed to programs that assured clean water supplies, uncontaminated food and more sanitary living arrangements. Most people, however, have very little idea of the job possibilities in this area. They see physicians, nurses and hospitals on television dramas. They get care from their own physicians but they rarely come in contact with those who work in providing preventive services.

In 1880, 90 percent of all surgical wounds became infected and at least 75 percent of all abdominal operations proved fatal. A hospital was a place where people went to die. Most physicians learned by apprenticeship, just as most carpenters or auto mechanics learn their trade today. Bleeding and vomiting were advocated as acceptable methods of treatment by some of the most prestigious early training centers. It wasn't until about 1910, as has been often noted, that an average patient seeking help from an average physician had a better than 50–50 chance of benefiting from the encounter.

Today, medicine is becoming more concerned with what it takes to keep people healthy rather than what it takes to cure them once they are sick. Concern has been placed on changing people's personal habits—lifestyle, smoking, drinking, eating, exercise—in order to improve their health and life expectancy. Slowly the priorities in the health sector are shifting and a new importance is being placed on those who provide preventive services.

Those who work to protect our health rather than to cure our illnesses are found in diverse and sometimes unexpected settings. At the present time, most of these workers are employed by public health agencies. There are local health departments that collect vital statistics, monitor the environment, inspect facilities and develop special preventive programs. State health departments provide support for these local efforts. At the national level, the Center for Disease Control, the National Center for Health Statistics, the Food and Drug Administration, the Occupational Health and Safety Administration and the Public Health Service are responsible for assisting in efforts to protect people's health. These efforts employ individuals with highly specialized, technical backgrounds as well as those with little in the way of technical education.

Jobs related to protecting people's health are increasing in other kinds of settings too. The meat and poultry inspector in chapter 16 is just one of the many preventive health workers behind the scenes who make sure that the food you eat, the house you live in, the air you breathe and the place where you work are safe. Health educators, such as the one introduced in chapter 15, work in community health centers, health system agencies and, increasingly, in hospitals. Their job is to make people more aware of what they can do to protect their own health. An individual such as the exercise physiologist in chapter 14 is a part of perhaps the most rapidly growing area in the health sector. In addition to the carefully controlled industrial exercise program that the exercise physiologist works with, there are a wide variety of people working in local Ys, health spas and with commercial and voluntary organizations. They assist people in changing their eating, smoking and exercise habits so they can live healthier, happier and more productive lives.

14

EXERCISE PHYSIOLOGIST

The corporate headquarters where Dan Radner works is tucked into a sheltered valley, back from the road. On the ridge, two hundred yards from the main building, is a fenced-in, flat asphalt surface with a white circle in the center. The company helicopter lands here, ferrying executives to and from the international airport. The large white cement building blends into the rolling pasture land around it. An inconspicuous sign marks the entrance. Just below the building is an irregularly shaped reflecting pond with a fountain in the middle.

Dan nods to the receptionist in the interior courtyard. The enclosed courtyard extends through the entire length of the building. Five floors of offices overlook it. Christmas is a couple of weeks away and the courtyard is filled with poinsettias.

Several men sitting in the red leather chairs in the courtyard smile and wave at Dan. Dan, though younger and taller, looks much like the two men he passes. He is wearing a dark, three-piece suit and carries a briefcase. His steel rim glasses and his mannerisms are those of a quiet, studious person. He is hardly the kind of person you would expect to have played offensive center for a professional football team.

Dan walks down the staircase to the lower level. The fitness program is located across from the executive dining area. Inside the stark white room with tan carpeting, the cleaning woman is just finishing up, polishing one of the gleaming white exercise bicycles. Along one wall are full-length mirrors and four red motor-driven treadmills, conveyor belts surrounded by metal bars to help a person maintain his position. Along the other wall are two gold colored rowing machines. A row of dumbells and a large blue exercise machine complete the assortment of equipment in the room.

Dan's small, windowless office is off to the side of the exercise room. He sits down at the desk and checks over his schedule.

"We run the fitness center on a flexible basis. Some of our clients like to come in early in the morning before work, others late in the evening, so we try to accommodate both. On Mondays, Wednesdays and Fridays we are open from seven to three. On Tuesdays and Thursdays we are open from eleven to seven in the evening. The majority of our clients like to exercise during the lunch hour, so this schedule accommodates them any day of the week."

"Excuse me, Mr. Radner, here's the Rolodex you asked for."

"Oh, hi Eleanor, yes that will be just fine." Dan takes the plastic address file from the secretary and places it on his desk. "Eleanor, we need to go over the list of those who will get the awards."

Eleanor nods and leaves.

"Since this is a corporate setting, we pay special attention to developing motivational tools. We are awarding certificates and patches from the President's Council on Physical Fitness to those participants completing the distance requirements in such activities as jogging and cycling. We are dealing with a very competitive group of people here and you'd be surprised how well incentives such as these work. Just carrying around a gym bag in this complex has become a real status symbol. If we give the awards to the right people, the ones that are real trend setters, we know that just about everybody here will want one too.

"I'm not an employee of this corporation. I'm part of a company that markets coronary diagnostic, preventive and rehabilitative services to corporations. We have a contract here to provide a program. It makes sense for this corporation because we have a number of specialized consultants, cardiologists and so forth that we can call in. If they just hired one person on their own to run a program for them, they wouldn't have this kind of expert assistance. We just started offering this service to corporations last year and we already have several contracts.

"I think this field is going to take off very quickly. We can market our programs to companies as a cost effective benefits package. We think the program more than pays for itself. The President's Council on Physical Fitness estimates that more than $7 billion is paid out each year by companies in the form of insurance benefits for people who die or are disabled prematurely as the result of heart attacks. A generally accepted rule of thumb in business is that your executive's net worth to the company is about five times his annual salary. That's what it costs the company to pay benefits to his widow, replace him and absorb the cost of bad decisions that will be made until his replacement has developed sufficient experience. You don't easily replace a person who has twenty to thirty years experience. So, our program will be cost effective if we can just prevent a few of those premature deaths. There is going to be a growing demand for these kinds of services.

"Our major objective is to reduce the risk of a person having a coronary. If a person has high blood pressure, high serum cholesterol levels, high serum triglyceride levels, is overweight, smokes, is physically inactive, faces an inordinate amount of emotional stress in day to day life or has a family history of heart attacks, she or he is a high risk candidate for a heart attack. The only risk factors we can't change through our prescriptive exercise program is the individual's heredity. Everything else we're usually successful in reducing."

Dan leans back in his chair, stretches and smiles.

"It's funny how I got into this area. I majored in philosophy in college. Athletics was the other part of my life. I played football, wrestled, was on the rowing team, and I got a great deal of enjoyment out of all these things. After I had been out of school a couple of years, I decided I wanted to go into medicine. I went back and got a second undergraduate degree in biology with a minor in chemistry, but I didn't make it into medical school. I didn't want to give up all I had invested, so I started looking for a related area. I entered a graduate program in exercise physiology and started to seriously study the effects of exercise on the human body. It seemed a perfect way to combine all of my interests.

"There's still a stigma attached to the whole area of exercise physiology, though. Most people still think of us as gym teachers in tight T-shirts and whistles who toss out basketballs. It's only in the last few years that the profession has moved out of the rah, rah jock stage and into serious science. Looking at the biochemical and cardiological impact of exercise is a new development. The traditional medical approach has been to look at the pathology of isolated organs in the resting state as opposed to the dynamic state. People who had had heart attacks would go to their cardiologist and ask about exercise and she or he would say 'yeah, exercise,' but neither of them would have a clear idea of what that meant. The exercise physiology approach looks at the impact of exercise on organs. It's only recently that the benefits of exercise on the cardiovascular system have been scientifically proven. We now know fairly precisely what has to be done to reduce a person's risk of having a heart attack and how to rehabilitate a person who has had one.

"Exercise helps do three things that reduce the chance of a heart attack. First, it helps increase the flow of blood to and from the heart by developing stronger contractile properties in the heart muscle. That is, each beat is more efficient and the heart doesn't have to beat as frequently. That's why the pulse rate for long distance runners is so much lower than for the average person. Another thing that happens is that the number and size of the coronary capillaries increase."

Dan turns and points to a round-shaped object embedded in a plastic cube on his desk.

"This is a latex perfused cow's heart. The white lines running through it are capillaries. They carry blood to the heart muscle and provide it with oxygen. When these get blocked you start having problems.

"Finally, there are some very important biochemical changes that take place with exercise. The absolute level of triglycerides in the blood is reduced and the proportion of low density to high density lipoproteins in the cholesterol is also reduced. Both of these changes appear to reduce the risk of a heart attack. High triglyceride levels and a high proportion of low density lipoproteins in the serum apparently contribute to the production of placque in the arteries. That results in hardening of the arteries and, eventually, complete blockage of the artery. That's when you have a heart attack. Before that happens a person may have some warning signs in terms of angina (chest pains), sort of mini crises resulting from the heart not getting sufficient oxygen.

"After my first year of graduate school, I started working at a heart clinic. It was a free standing clinic that helped heart attack victims or those who had had heart surgery. There is a growing number of people around who have had open heart surgery.

They've formed a group called the Zipper Club. That's because those who have heart surgery have a zipper-like scar down the middle of their chest. The Club provides support and counseling to its members. The heart clinic worked with them in a rehabilitative capacity. You see, the problem with a heart attack victim is that a person either becomes a 'cardiac cripple,' paralyzed by fear and unwilling to do anything, or the person just plows ahead and goes back to all of her or his normal activities. Both of these alternatives are completely unacceptable. The clinic was set up to develop a rational means for rehabilitating the heart patient. It was staffed by cardiologists, nurses and exercise physiologists. The exercise physiologists were the newcomers to the health care fraternity but the cardiologists and the nurses learned to trust us and appreciate what we were able to offer. You see, the physical therapist only works on joints and muscles. Once a person has achieved a certain range of motion, that's where it ends. The heart, however, is a hidden muscle and it's not quite as easy to determine how much strength it has or how to increase its strength and efficiency. That's where we came into the picture. We'd help to evaluate stress tests, design exercise programs for the clinic's patients and keep careful tabs on their progress.

"I went from there to working with our new company. Our first contract was with this corporation.

"Each of the executives in this complex gets a comprehensive annual physical by Dr. Johnson, the company physician. He knows most of them very well and has been the personal physician to many of them for years. Dr. Johnson refers people to our program. They're either individuals that he considers at high coronary risk or people who have enough clout in the organization to persuade him to let them in. The company has decided to restrict entry into the program. We know the ones we get are going to be serious and highly motivated to stick with the program. It's important to keep a high level of participation in the program. Too many dropouts would be interpreted as a sign of a lack of interest.

"Each person, before starting in our prescriptive exercise program, must have a complete physical workup. We pay particular attention to the blood work. A pulmonary function test (a test of lung capacity) and a cardiovascular stress test (a test of the effect of various levels of exercise on the heart) are also performed.

"After the entire workup is complete, we sit down with the individual and discuss the objectives of the program. We do a coronary risk factor workup and explain it to them. The primary goal of the program is to lower the participant's risk of heart attack, but we also include goals that each individual has. This helps to keep them motivated. A person might like to improve her or his tennis or golf game and we can devise exercises that will help an individual do that.

"The next step is to take baseline physiological measures on the actual exercise equipment we will be using. We take their blood pressure and pulse after using each of the types of equipment we have. Using these baseline measures, we develop an individualized exercise prescription.

"There are three phases to an exercise session. There's a warm-up phase where we prescribe bending and stretching exercises to increase heart rate and prepare them for the working phase. The next phase is the working portion of the session. We have what we call a circuit interval exercise system. We alternate exercises that put heavy stress on the person's heart, such as the treadmill, the bicycle and the rowing machines, with isotonic, muscle building exercises, such as situps, bench presses and so forth. Even though these isotonic exercises are real work, they don't put much stress on the heart. As a result, by alternating these two kinds of exercises, we can maintain a person's heart rate at close to what we've determined should be the optimal rate. We keep a close watch on them during the first six months and take their blood pressure readings at least three times during every exercise session.

"We want them to schedule at least three visits a week. Each exercise session takes approximately an hour to complete. All of these men are pressed for time and have appointments scheduled every fifteen minutes. We have their secretaries block out the exercise times for them. This has been really helpful in keeping their attendance up. The secretaries commit them to coming to the exercise program and won't schedule any meetings that conflict with those times."

"We haven't had much trouble with attendance though. One thing about top executives is that when they commit themselves to doing something, they do it. Maybe not for the right reasons, maybe they're driven, competitive, compulsive or whatever, but they do it."

"Excuse me, is anybody in the women's locker room?" The janitor sticks his head into Dan's office.

"No, it's all clear, go ahead." Dan smiles. "We have one woman in the program. Since our program is aimed at reducing cardiac risks, it's mostly designed for men. Heart attacks, at least up to now, have been pretty much a health problem for males. Up until age thirty-five neither men nor women are interested in an exercise program other than for its cosmetic effects. After age thirty-five, men start becoming concerned about their hearts."

Dan points to a stack of video tape cartridges in the corner of his office. "We try to make it as pleasant for people to participate as possible. We have all of the tapes of Bronowski's "Ascent of Man" television series. They can watch the tapes on a color television screen while they exercise. It helps to combat boredom. These executives are all 'type A' people, always concerned with packing as much into a day as possible, and feeling pressured for time. They tend to engage in polyphasic thinking, doing and thinking about more than one thing at a time.

"We stress to them that it takes about six weeks before there are any training effects, that is, greater pulmonary and cardiovascular efficiency. However, it takes only two weeks to lose it all. If any of our people go away, and many of them travel a great deal, we design an exercise maintenance program for them to take with them. Even if they have no other place to do it, they can maintain their conditioning by jogging in place and doing certain prescribed exercises in their hotel room.

"At the end of six months they're tested again and we schedule an hour with each of them to discuss the results. We explain what changes have taken place in their heart rate under physical stress, their blood pressure, the change in the amount of body fat they have and so forth. We also try to determine how they feel about the program. We counsel them on diet, if they need to lose weight, and we talk to them about their smoking habits. Their drinking is a sensitive area, but we try to help those who are perhaps doing a little too much. We try to give them a comprehensive idea of where they are in terms of their overall health. In general, those who have stuck with the program and exercised at least three times a week show marked improvement."

"Hi, Dan." A man waves from across the exercise room. He grabs a key and disappears into the locker room. A few minutes later he emerges in white tennis shorts and a blue tennis top. He takes his exercise card out of the file next to where the locker keys are hung and sticks it on a clipboard. He then begins to warm up, humming to himself. He has balding, white hair and a bit of a paunch.

Dan puts on the white laboratory coat that's hanging next to his desk and stuffs a stethoscope into his pocket.

"Hi, John, are you ready to go to work on the treadmill?"

John nods.

"All right, let me get you set up. Remember, get on the treadmill one foot at a time." Dan takes the clipboard from John, checks the prescription and adjusts the speed of the treadmill. "Call me when the timer gets to five minutes, John. I want to be sure to get a reading on you."

"One of the most important things about this program is the precautions we take. We watch the participants very closely. We are trained in CPR (cardiopulmonary resuscitation) and we have a defibrillator in the supply room, just in case. We also have direct, immediate communication with security. They'll get an ambulance here as soon as possible. The company doctor is on call at all times that we're open. We have developed all of these elaborate precautions even though we've never had to use them. It helps make our participants feel comfortable. One told me the other day that what he really liked about the program was the sense of security. He was afraid to start exercising on his own."

"Dan, I'm just about there," calls John, who has been walking at a fast pace on the treadmill. Dan walks over and puts the blood pressure cuff on him while John continues walking on the treadmill.

"OK, John," Dan makes a note on the exercise card and hands the clipboard back to him.

Two other men enter the exercise room, grab locker keys, and return dressed in tennis shorts.

"Hey John, how you doing?" one of them calls. The two begin their warm-up exercises. John has moved on to the rowing machine. The two newcomers, who have been in the program longer than John, make their own, faster settings on the treadmills and hop on. Dan stands close by, waiting to take blood pressure readings. The two start jogging on the treadmills, staring at themselves in the floor-length mirror in front of them.

"The nice thing about treadmills is that even though they're set at different speeds, nobody passes you. These men are really competitive. If you had a track, one of them would start lapping the others, it would drive them crazy. They'd try to kill themselves keeping up and they'd probably never come back. They'd feel too humiliated. With the treadmills, everybody goes at their own pace and nobody feels that the others are getting ahead of them."

"Dan, would you put one of those tapes on for me," one of them calls.

Dan inserts one of the video cassettes into the tape deck and wheels the television into position next to the treadmill. The two continue to jog to the thoughtful introduction of Bronowski.

"Some of these men live under real pressure. John, for example, is involved in some of the key decisions. The wrong one could mean the loss of millions of dollars."

Three younger men in business suits poke their heads in the door of the exercise room. They stare at the equipment in the room. They appear impressed.

The man who asked for the video tape has just begun the cooling down phase. He is loudly humming the tune coming from the video tape, swinging two dumbells back and forth.

"Catch you for lunch, Harry?" John calls to him on the way to the locker room.

"Sure, John, I'll be through in a few minutes," Harry says.

After all three have left, Dan checks their exercise cards. He changes the prescription on John's card so that he will have to work a little harder while on the treadmill during his next exercise session. He leaves the other two at the same level and refiles the cards.

"It's funny, there is very little shop talk in the exercise room. Mostly they talk about political happenings or social engagements. That's good. We want them to see it as a respite from their work day, not just a part of it.

"There are a lot of special problems our participants have that we try to help them with. Most of them have problems with low back pain. Most people over fifty have problems with this. There are some specific exercises that are helpful. Some of our participants have knee problems that we can help them with. Hypertension, arthritis and obesity are some of the other chronic problems that we try to help our participants with.

"What most people don't realize before they get involved in

something like this is that it doesn't have to hurt to get results. In fact, you can get almost as much benefit out of an exercise program that involves moderate effort as you can from one that is totally exhausting."

Other men come and go through their exercise programs. The lunch crowd disappears around two and the exercise room is quiet for a while. Activity begins to pick up again around five.

"This whole field is in its infancy. It's going to grow rapidly. People have become much more health conscious and we're beginning to know what we need to do to help them. There's a void that we fill. Most physicians need assistance in designing exercise prescriptions for their patients. There's a need for people who are really qualified in the exercise area. They're going to need academic credentials and they'll need to present themselves as professionals. We have to move away from the "jock" stigma. I don't think that an undergraduate degree is sufficient. I think a good pre-med undergraduate background and a master's program where you're really taught to think is essential. People who have been involved in athletics and who have good undergraduate science backgrounds are good potential recruits for exercise technicians. Program directors, however, are going to need extensive graduate training and clinical preparation. In addition, people coming into this field need to know how to deal with people and have adequate management skills. They need to know how to manage a budget and how to develop a program. There's no room for inadequately trained people. You're dealing with people's lives and you have to know exactly what you're doing. If somebody is overdoing it and you see their gait staggering you have to be there to catch it.

"We're just starting a credentialling program sponsored by the American College of Sports Medicine. Candidates will have to take a written, oral and practical clinical exam that will test their ability to write exercise prescriptions and supervise an exercise program. There will be an exam for program directors and for exercise technicians, who will work under the supervision of a program director. The program directors are the ones that will be required to hold a Ph.D or its equivalent, and I think that's where the emphasis should be placed right now.

"It's an attractive field to become involved in. The field is expanding. I plan eventually to move into more of a management position in our company, supervising program directors in a number of settings. Program directors are salaried between $10,000 and $40,000 depending on the size of their program and their ability to make the program a success. Of course, there are problems. As soon as a company comes on hard times, they may decide to eliminate their prescriptive exercise program. I don't think, however, that it poses an enormous problem to programs like this one which focus on the top executives. After all, they're the ones that make the budget cutting decisions and they're also the ones that directly benefit from the program." Dan laughs.

The last participant in the exercise program checks out a few minutes before seven and Dan locks up behind him. He waves to the security guard at the desk in the courtyard and heads for his car. It's dark. Only a few office lights in the building are still on. The day, for most of the executives who look after the health of the large corporation and for Dan, who looks after the health of the executives, is over.

SUMMARY

DUTIES: *Works in collaboration with an individual's physician to design and supervise an exercise program. Performs diagnostic tests, develops exercise prescriptions and monitors the results. Assumes responsibilities for the administration of such programs in rehabilitation centers, executive health programs, Ys and commercial health spas.*

TRAINING: *Undergraduate and master's degree programs in exercise physiology are available in a number of universities. There are national certification exams for program directors and exercise technicians. A master's degree is generally required for program directors and an undergraduate degree in exercise physiology is preferred for exercise technicians. For more information, contact:*

> *American College of Sports Medicine*
> *1440 Monroe Street*
> *Madison, Wisconsin   53706*

SALARY: *$10,000–40,000 depending on experience and responsibilities.*

15

HEALTH EDUCATOR

Bright sunshine lights the upper half of the old hospital entrance as Kathy Moore crosses the courtyard. The sedate hallway inside is quiet, insulated from the street traffic and from the faster pace of the new hospital, connected to the older building by a long corridor.

The old building was completed over one hundred years ago. It was recently refurbished and is now used only for offices. It includes some displays for visitors on how medicine was practiced in the nineteenth century. It is strange that such a building, so immersed in the past, should be heavily involved at the same time in community health education. Most hospitals view such activities with indifference, an unnecessary frill, something that isn't quite accepted. Yet, maybe it's not as strange as it seems. There was less reliance on physicians and hospitals then. Health education is an old idea that is getting new attention.

Kathy climbs two steps at a time up the large circular staircase to her third-floor office. She stops at the landing on the third floor to stare out across the courtyard toward the two newer hospital buildings.

"It's going to be a great fall weekend," she says. She is a small woman with short brown hair and a mischievous smile.

"Health education is a mixed bag," Kathy explains. "Everybody is involved in education. A lot of people don't understand the need for separate individuals who specialize in this area. Especially in hospitals, people are very sensitive about others infringing on their turf. A team approach is what is needed, but sometimes it's hard to get that across. Some doctors will tell you, 'My patients don't want any more information. I give them all they need to know. I won't let you near them with a ten foot pole.' It takes a while for the doctors to come around. Usually what happens is that a patient asks why she or he can't participate in our program when the person in the next bed, who has the same condition, can. The doctor may look into it and then realize how the program can help a patient understand her or his treatment.

"There are a lot of different people doing health education in different kinds of settings. Usually nurses have worked into these roles in hospitals. It sort of flows naturally from the kind of patient education that a nurse gets involved in anyway. Then, of course, you can't exclude those with physical education backgrounds who get involved in teaching health education in schools or in conducting exercise and weight watching classes in Ys and health spas. The large voluntary agencies, like the heart association, have television spots that focus on getting information to people about certain health problems they may have. But you have to be careful about that stuff. You can give people information, but to really educate them means that you change their behavior. I think, at least as far as health behavior is concerned, that takes a little more than just some television spots. There are also master's degree programs in health education in schools of public health. Health education has been done for a long time by health departments, particularly for such problems as VD and lead poisoning. Hospitals have been slow in getting involved."

Kathy was trained as a nurse. She went through a three-year hospital diploma program. "It was a choice between going to college and becoming a teacher, going to nursing school or becoming a secretary. I went to the nursing school because it didn't cost as much as four years of college and I couldn't handle being a secretary," she explains.

"It's funny. I've been a diabetic since I was nine. I never thought of myself as being sick. I guess my mother was really good for me. She let me know that I'd pretty much have to take care of myself. It wasn't that she wasn't concerned, just that she knew it was better not to hover over me. I've seen some kids with diabetes who have really been messed up in that way by their families. Anyway, I just applied to nursing school, taking for granted I'd get in. I was a pretty good student in high school. It was only after I'd been there a year that the dean called me in and explained that I almost hadn't been admitted. I was the first student with diabetes they had considered and they weren't sure whether they should admit me. They said I had set a good precedent and they had decided to admit another student for the next year. They wanted me to look after her. Thank goodness she wasn't the first they admitted. She was terrible! Always going on eating binges and getting sick. She just had never learned to take care of herself.

"I worked as a nurse on a hospital floor for a couple of years and then worked my way through a pre-med science program as a school nurse. It was rough, classes, nights in the school infirmary and weekends working in a hospital back home, but I made it. Got admitted to a medical school finally too. But then it just seemed like too much to think about another four to six years of school and unfortunately, my brother was killed in Vietnam about that time. I got a job doing research in diabetes and helped teach diabetics care to patients in a medical school clinic. It helped to combine most of my interests. It wasn't long till I got into the education full time. I worked for a year for the Diabetes Association developing programs. Then I worked as a health education project director in a hospital.

"I got this job five months ago. I mean these surroundings. I just didn't believe it at first," she gazes at the high ceilings and spacious arched windows in her office. "I get a lot of support from administration, which can be a problem in many hospitals. They're committed to health education here. In most hospitals, since it's not reimbursable, other things have higher priority.

"A lot of people argue about where health education should take place. They say that a hospital is the wrong place, too concerned with curing people rather than preventing illness. Schools and health departments should do it along with the voluntary agencies like the Heart Association. Well, some of these groups do a good job, but that shouldn't exclude the hospital from getting involved too. I see the hospital as a school for community health education. We have a lot of resources and expertise. One real advantage is that the people who come here, the patients and their families, are really motivated to learn something about taking care of themselves. It's an excellent place for such education. We try to determine what is needed by our inpatients, outpatients, by our employees and by the general community, however you define it."

Kathy waves her hand at the window.

"Everybody in a hospital is involved in health education. Health educators help it happen, encourage it, point out where it is needed, provide the resources and technical assistance to staff members who are interested.

"When I got here the first thing I tried to do was to collect some materials that others would need for teaching about health. I could say, 'Here's something we can offer you now.' "

The large tables in the room are stacked with different colored pamphlets, tape cassettes and training films. Her large new office is already beginning to look crowded.

"People on the staff need help getting their educational programs down on paper, identifying the objectives they want. I try to help. Right now, I'm still in the process of identifying needs. We've got some programs going already and our activities are going to pick up quickly this fall. Let's see, there's a group of volunteers that will be here at ten. We have a very active group of volunteers. In fact, Helen and Mary really help make this program work."

Helen, Kathy's assistant, has been working quietly on the other side of the room putting packets of materials together. She looks up and smiles.

"Helen, I'm going to grab some coffee before that group comes in. If they come early, show them where we're going to be."

Kathy jogs down the circular stairs.

"Hospital politics and coffee," Kathy smiles. "The cafeteria is where everything gets decided. Somehow it's easier to meet people there. You can get a lot of things ironed out. People are more relaxed . . . it's kind of neutral turf."

Nancy, the director of Inservice Education, is in the line just ahead of Kathy. They grab coffee and donuts and hunt for a quiet corner. Nurses and several doctors in green surgical garb sit at the table opposite them. A few patients in robes sit quietly by themselves, but most of the tables are filled with nurses, medical residents and interns. They have to lean toward each other to be heard above the din.

"We've started a CPR (cardiopulmonary resuscitation) course for the staff," Kathy says. "That's one way to get the bugs out of the program before we open it up to the general public."

"My secretary is taking the course," Nancy says. "She came in this morning saying, 'Oh, I'm so stiff.' "

The participants had practiced getting a heart started again through external massage. Life-like inflated manikins are used. It can be a workout for someone not used to exercise.

"We try to keep the classes informal," Kathy explains. "A lot of people are scared to death of classrooms, people who have been housekeepers or aides and out of school for a long time. They freeze up. We try to keep the classes small and informal and keep the language as non-technical as possible. Those of us who have worked a long time in health care forget the special language we develop. People will sit there while you talk away. They may not understand a thing you've said, but they'll nod and smile the whole time. You have to be careful."

Nancy nodded in agreement. "We just finished an inservice course on 'touching.' You know, how to touch when it is helpful to touch someone, when it is harmful, that sort of thing. We had the same course for the aides and the nurses, but the language we used in each was completely different."

"Frank, from the security office here, told me that George complained this morning after the CPR class of sore lips," Kathy says.

"Boy, I don't know what that will do to the classes if it gets around," Nancy smiles.

"Well, you ought to help spread that rumor. We're sure to get a long waiting list for the classes," Kathy says.

They both laugh.

The CPR programs are a joint effort of the hospital's education and respiratory therapy departments. The course is taught in five sessions. So far, the instructors have been volunteers from within the hospital. Soon they will get a fee for each course. The course will be offered next to people in the community.

"You have to go very slowly and carefully through it and give everybody plenty of practice so that they can do it perfectly. In a real situation, you're sure to miss some of the things, so we want to make sure that people really get it down . . . make it all pretty automatic."

They talk more about how to recruit staff for the inservice course and then Kathy talks about some of the other projects that are starting up.

"I'm working with the nursing department right now. They want to start a program so that every woman who comes into the hospital is taught how to do a breast self-examination. They really want to push it."

"We're also going to set up a series of programs at the YMCA for senior citizens," Kathy says. "We'll have discussions of vision, arthritis, foot-care and diabetes."

The coffee finished, Kathy has to get back to the meeting with the volunteers.

"Keep me posted on what we can do to help out in putting together some programs," Kathy says.

Nancy smiles and waves.

The volunteers have already assembled in the small classroom. Kathy gives them a short talk about what health education is about.

"Health education may be kind of a scary word. You may feel it doesn't have anything to do with you, but we're all involved in health education. Most of the time, we must be our own doctors. Even if you see a doctor every other week and you're fortunate enough to see him for a half hour each time, well, that's still only twelve hours a year and the rest of the time you're on your own. What you do and don't do will help you stay well. It's mainly your responsibility."

She explains the various programs that will be available to them. "We're offering a smoking cessation program. It works and the cost is minimal. You can also join our CPR classes that are starting this fall. We're going to keep the classes small because we want to make sure everybody in the class learns the techniques perfectly."

"The other thing that you should be aware of is the TelMed program that we've started. We have a library of taped health information. People can call and request to listen to a tape by telephone. There are pamphlets here that tell about it. Feel free to use it. Also, we need volunteers to help at the switchboard. We're very much dependent on volunteers to make the program work and we're counting on you."

The volunteers see a video tape on the history of the hospital. They enjoy the presentation and mutter approval to themselves. There are some senior citizens, some high-school students and some housewives in the group.

Kathy returns to her office. Two people from the education department of a hospital in a neighboring state have come to learn about the TelMed program. Together, Kathy and her visitors walk over to the adjoining building where the switchboards are located.

The visitors are interested in setting up a system in their hospital similar to the one developed in Kathy's hospital. The idea originated with the San Bernardino Medical Society in California and now there are TelMed centers in seventy-five different locations across the country. The hospital gets 700 to 1,400 calls a week. There are close to two hundred taped messages. They provide a caller with information on birth control, care of children, drug problems, acne, dandruff, sore throats, getting ready for the skiing season—all the most commonly asked questions about health and health care.

"One of the things you have to think about, particularly if you're going to use volunteers," Kathy tells her guests, "is where you locate the switchboards. A lot of the volunteers are senior citizens and they have some trouble making it up the stairs to where we have the unit now. They are also fearful about working in the evening."

The two switchboards are located on the second floor of the adjoining building. Each switchboard can handle up to twenty calls at a time. The tape library surrounds the telephone console. When Kathy and her guests arrive, the supervisor leaves the console to greet them.

"How's it going, Betty?" Kathy asks.

"Oh, it was slow this morning, but it's beginning to pick up. I got a call from a woman a few minutes ago. She wanted to hear the tape 'No-No–What Does It Mean to the Toddler?' I could barely hear her over the screams of the child in the background."

They all laugh.

Kathy spends a few more minutes answering questions.

"Sorry, I'm going to have to rush off and attend to some other things. There's a good deli down the street a couple of blocks, if you want some lunch. Good luck to you both. If you think of any other questions later, give me a call."

The two guests thank her at the door and Kathy waves good-bye as she heads back to her office. She grabs a sandwich from the hospital cafeteria and picks up her mail on the way. Some of the training films she ordered have arrived. Back in her office she orders some stroke pamphlets for one of the nursing supervisors. Around two o'clock she leaves her paper work to run errands.

It takes fifteen minutes by car to cover the short distance to the Red Cross.

"The Red Cross manages some of the CPR training in the city.

The rest is done by the Heart Association. I need to borrow some more manikins from The Red Cross for next week's classes and ask about some additional funds for expanding the program. Gosh, I hope I don't get a ticket."

She squeezes into a No Parking space next to the corner of the curb. The Red Cross offices are on one of the top floors of a bank building. Kathy takes the elevator to the appropriate floor. The secretary in the carpeted reception area looks up and smiles.

"Janet's office is over on the left. She's expecting you."

Janet rises from her desk as Kathy enters.

"Hi," Kathy says. "It's good to have a chance to meet face-to-face, finally."

Janet smiles. "I guess you want to borrow those two fellows." She points to two large suitcases in the corner of the room.

"Great, how long can we have them?"

"Oh, we don't have any other plans for them right now. Keep them till the end of the program."

They talk about future plans for the city's CPR program. Kathy's group will play a major role.

"Hey, let me get John to help you carry these two guys down to your car. They're heavy."

John, a husky six-footer, follows Kathy into the elevator with one of the suitcases under each arm.

A policeman is writing out a ticket on the car next to hers. He pauses and stares at them as they stuff the two coffin-sized suitcases in the back seat.

"Whew, that was close." Kathy laughs, as she pulls out into the traffic.

She stops by the Heart Association on her way back to the hospital. It's a large remodeled home with old wooden floors.

"I need to get some pamphlets for the folder we give out in the CPR course. There's one on the anatomy and physiology of the heart and one about CPR techniques that they can take home and review. There is also a questionnaire they can fill out to score their own risks of getting a heart attack. Smoking, exercise patterns, changing homes or jobs—all of those things increase your chances of getting a heart attack. We include a pamphlet on the TelMed program too, since there are four or five tapes that they may want to listen to about heart attacks."

Kathy sits down and has a cup of coffee with Bob and Marilyn, two staff people at the Heart Association. They talk about the progress of the CPR program. Bob and Marilyn were trained as social workers, but they too are working mostly in health education.

After talking for a while, Kathy gathers up the box of pamphlets she needs and heads for her car.

"It's good to get out and see the people in these agencies. It helps in working with them later. I suppose I could send one of the volunteers on these kinds of errands, but it's really an excuse to start getting acquainted."

Arriving back at the hospital, she unloads the manikins and literature at the loading dock. Ron, one of the maintenance workers, agrees to take the things to her office.

When Kathy returns to her office, it is almost time to go home. Mary, the afternoon volunteer, has just finished showing a video tape to a lung patient. The patient is a thin, pale man with white hair. His wife, a heavyset woman with glasses and a flowered dress, is holding his hand. They ask several questions about the tape they have just seen, thank Kathy and Mary and leave.

"Thanks for helping out, Mary," Kathy says.

"Have a nice weekend," Mary says, as she pulls on her coat to go.

Kathy sorts through the afternoon mail on her desk. Everything is set for next week. She takes one more quick check of the materials in her office and then also escapes into the warm, autumn sunshine.

SUMMARY

DUTIES: *Develops health education programs for health departments, hospitals or voluntary associations. This involves identifying educational needs, designing programs to meet those needs and evaluating the results. Some are employed by elementary and high schools to teach health education.*

TRAINING: *A master's in health education from a school of public health is helpful, although many who work in this field do not have one. Nurses usually assume responsibility for most of the health education that goes on in hospitals. For information on public health education training programs, contact:*

> *American Public Health Association*
> *1015 18th Street NW*
> *Washington, D.C. 20036*

For information on hospital-based community health education, contact:

> *Office of Consumer Health Education*
> *College of Medicine and Dentistry of New Jersey*
> *Rutgers Medical School*
> *Piscataway, New Jersey 08854*

SALARY: *$12,000–30,000 depending on experience and responsibilities.*

16

U.S.D.A.
MEAT AND POULTRY
INSPECTOR

There would be meat that had tumbled out on the floor in the dirt and the sawdust, where the workers had tramped and spit uncounted billions of consumption germs. There would be meat stored in great piles in rooms and the water from the leaky roofs would drip over it, and thousands of rats would race about on it. It was too dark in these storage spaces to see well, but a man could run his hands over these piles of meat and sweep off handsful of dried dung of rats ... There were the butt ends of smoked meat and the scraps of corned beef and all the odds and ends that would be dumped into barrels in the cellar and left there. Under the system of rigid economy ... some jobs ... it only paid to do once in a long time. Among these was cleaning out the waste barrels. Every spring they did it, and in the barrels would be dirt and rust and old nails and staled water and cartload after cartload of it would be taken up and dumped into the hoppers with fresh meat and sent out to the public's breakfast ... (*The Jungle*, Upton Sinclair, 1905, p. 135, Robert Bentley, Inc.)

The whine of diesel engines and the flash of headlights from the livestock trucks pierce the early morning fog at the gates to Gorham Foods. A guard beckons the trucks through, one by one. Inside the yards, a row of unloading docks waits to receive the animals from the semis and the farm pick-ups that stream into Gorham throughout the day. They come with sheep, cattle and hogs to one of the largest meat processing plants in the world.

Parts of the Gorham food plant are over a hundred years old. Much of it is painted brick and the buildings have many narrow stairs and small windows. Dr. Sam McDonnell has an office on the second floor with a window overlooking the unloading area. A big white sign with red letters faces his window from the unloading sheds, *Livestock Bruise Easily. Handle Them Carefully!* Dr.

U.S.D.A. MEAT AND POULTRY INSPECTOR

McDonnell, a veterinarian, is the inspector in charge of the United States Department of Agriculture (U.S.D.A.) meat inspection program at the Gorham plant.

"Things have changed a lot since Sinclair wrote that book, *The Jungle*," Dr. McDonnell says. He is in his early fifties and has been at the Gorham plant for the twelve years since he left private practice. "Oh yes, it was probably pretty true, what was in Sinclair's book. The first effective meat inspection laws were passed around 1906, and things have gotten more and more strict since then. But it doesn't happen without on-site inspection. There is a basic conflict, I'm afraid. Making a little more profit means cutting corners which often means lower product standards. Things usually go smoothly here. When the company is tight financially, you can feel the rub. We get a lot more complaints from the company during those times."

The meat and poultry inspection team is part of the federal system. Some states have their own teams that inspect facilities that are not involved in interstate commerce. Every animal that goes through the Gorham plant is inspected by Dr. McDonnell's team, both before and after slaughter. At the Gorham plant, this means 6,500 hogs, 1,100 cattle and 1,200 sheep per day.

"Gorham can't move meat out of the state without our team being here, not out of the state or out of the country. We have forty inspectors at this plant. Every step of production is inspected by our people, right from the time they unload the animals," Dr. McDonnell gestures toward the window, "until the bologna, hams and cold cuts move out.

"We have what we call our food inspectors, and then we have the supervising veterinarians. With the food inspectors we look primarily for someone with experience with livestock or meat operations, rather than formal education. Our food inspectors don't absolutely have to have a high-school diploma. They take a civil service test, and when an opening occurs they get on-the-job training and then go through a special course in Texas. That course takes a month and then they are assigned to a regular position.

"Everything we do here comes from these two books." Dr. McDonnell reaches for two large spiral bound volumes on his book shelf. "This is our book of regulations," he pats one. "That has the laws of meat inspection. And this other one is the interpretation and extension of the law. It tells us what procedures to follow to implement the law.

"I do get upset sometimes. We get criticism about not doing our work. But every one of the inspectors has a job to do out there, and they do it all day long. There's not much time for chitchat with 700 hogs going through here every hour."

Dr. Dan Smith is in the office with Dr. McDonnell. He is the veterinarian in the hog kill area. He is a tall slender man in his late thirties. At his main station he does the final inspection of carcasses for lesions from disease and other abnormalities. Depending on his verdict, the carcasses are either sent on to the cooler to be cut up the next day, or condemned as unfit for human food. This morning he is on his way down to the area where the hogs are killed to get a blood sample. The sample will be used to test for swine pseudo-rabies.

"Pseudo-rabies is a fairly new problem," Dr. Smith explains as he leaves the U.S.D.A. office and begins the winding trip to the kill. "We just got a new notice from the main office today. They tell us how often to sample. It's an effort to track down infected herds and stop the spread of the disease." He reaches an outside door and crosses an alley into a building with three stories rising above it.

Inside the building, the noise from machinery makes conversation impossible. Through a corridor, in the pounding noise, Dr. Smith carefully steps across a narrow channel of blood and up to the platform where the hogs are slaughtered. The live pigs arrive on a V-shaped conveyor from a flight below. As they reach the top, a big man in a T-shirt places the electric stunning device, one probe on the head and the other further down the spine. The stunned hog is dumped on a moving counter. A second man thrusts a pointed knife in the throat and dark blood spurts across the counter. A third man shackles the hind legs and the hog is lifted up onto the moving rail. The ride is up three flights to the room where the animals are cleaned and prepared for cutting. The sloping floor beneath the carcasses is a sheet of blood. Sunlight filters in dimly from high windows as the swinging line of hogs moves up.

Dr. Smith mouths an explanation to the stick man who nods. Only the squeals of the hogs rise above the noise of the machinery. When the next pig is stuck, Dr. Smith reaches toward the dark spurting blood with an open test tube, and fills it.

Crossing back to the main building, Dr. Smith explains the stunning.

"The law says the animals must be killed in a humane manner. They are not to suffer. With hogs, we use electric shock. They have to be alive when they are stuck in order to get a good bleed. When they started using this particular stunning device, they had some problems. The second probe was too far down on the spine and the hogs would snap their backs when they went out. With cattle, electric shock is too unpredictable. With the range of weights we get, a uniform shock would kill some of them and leave others tearing around. They use a captive bolt on them, shot from a special gun. You can take the animal out to see if it revives if you suspect the devices aren't working properly."

Back in the roar of the dressing area, Dr. Smith points out the procedures that go into cleaning the hogs: a run through a scalding tank, through a dehairing machine, then scrubbing brushes and flaming torches to remove more hair. Then they go past a line of Gorham employees. These employees stand on high metal platforms in order to reach the hogs as they move by on the rail. There are shavers who take off any remaining hair and head droppers who drop the head for inspection by the U.S.D.A. head inspectors.

Larry Jordan is one of the head inspectors. He has been at the plant for five years. His training was done in Omaha before the school was moved to Texas. Like the workers on the rail, Larry carries a knife and knife sharpeners in a scabbard on a stainless-steel chain belt. Behind him at the station is a knife sterilizer with 180° water and towels.

Larry and the other head inspectors look for signs of jaundice, tuberculosis, lymphoma and many other abnormal conditions in the glands of the head and neck. Any suspect animals are tagged. The tags are placed to show that they came from the head inspection station. Eventually the suspect animal goes to the finalizing area to be examined by Dr. Smith. He will decide whether the animals should pass, pass with restriction, or be marked condemned and not for use as human food. The condemned carcasses are cooked at high temperatures and are used as hog feed protein supplements. The rendered oils are used in soap making. Carcasses passed with restriction usually have to be used in a ground-up cooked product.

Ann Parker is further up the line on what is called the "viscera table." Ann is in her forties and only completed the special training in Texas six months ago. Her station comes right after the hogs have their internal organs removed. The viscera, or organs, from each carcass are placed in a shallow pan that moves along a conveyor belt parallel with the rail. Each pan is identified with its carcass. Ann's job is to inspect the pans of viscera as they move along in front of her. She pays particular attention to various lymph nodes, the liver and the heart. She dips her hands into a pan and checks the liver out quickly, folding it over, feeling for lesions and lumps, looking for spots and abnormal coloring. She also spreads the intestines to feel the lymph nodes in the membrane. If there are abnormalities she will stamp the organ in question. Occasionally an intestine will break open into the pan. Then she quickly stamps the whole pan "condemned," the blue marker slapping into the wetness.

"Some people would say this is disgusting," she shouts cheerfully above the noise. She is a neat woman with short curled hair. "But really, you get used to it. I'm still learning a lot and I get behind, but they . . ." she gestures to her two fellow inspectors, "they keep up on things for me. I think this work is important. My husband just didn't believe it when I told him we inspect every single hog that comes through here."

Beneath the work platform, men in raincoats and hard hats move along the cement floor, sweeping away the trimmings and blood. An inspector pushes a red button and the rail stops for some contamination to be trimmed off a carcass.

"Some people have to wait years to get into the inspection program," Ann says. "I was lucky. I signed up at a time when they needed people and I got in right away. We were in Texas for three weeks. They kept us real busy. You learn the whole process—live inspection, viscera, marking, grading, storage. We also learn about personal conduct on the job—things like misuse of property, acceptance of gifts, potential conflict in outside jobs—things like that."

Dr. Smith is back at his station, looking at suspect carcasses before they go to be cut up. Three carcasses have been detoured off the rail to his station. Their corresponding pans of viscera are there as well. One of the carcasses is yellow with advanced jaundice.

Dr. Smith stamps it "condemned, inedible." The other two have minor imperfections. Dr. Smith checks the viscera for signs of more advanced disease and then passes them.

"Of course, one of the big things with hogs was always trichinosis," Dr. Smith says. "Now we just assume that all hogs have some trichina. In fact, only a fraction of a percent do. But our legal assumption is that the consumer knows of the danger in fresh pork and will cook it thoroughly.

"Our job is to insure a safe, clean, wholesome product for the consumer. Part of this has to do with disease hazards. But it also has to do with having a pleasing product. Bruises in the meat aren't dangerous from a health standpoint, but they aren't very appealing to the eye.

"The emphasis in our work changes from time to time. The most difficult regulations to cope with have been those concerning chemical residues in meat. Right now, our big concern is with sulfa. The farmers are supposed to take their animals off sulfa drugs two weeks before slaughter. But it's tough on them. Sometimes the market prices will go up suddenly, and the temptation to bring in animals early is too great. Or sometimes you'll have a feed salesman who hasn't told the farmer about the sulfa withdrawal period. That's really hard. We test by the schedule we're sent from the area office. If we find animals with sulfa, we'll send them on through, but we'll trace them through the tattoos to the individual farmer or buying station. The next time that farmer sells here, the animals are bought conditionally and more samples are taken. If the residue is still in the carcass meat, the carcass is condemned.

"We don't often get direct contact with the sellers. Not too long ago we had a fellow bring in a hog that could hardly walk. His veterinarian had told him the hog had a pinched nerve or something. Well, Gorham will only buy a hog like that conditionally. The hog went through the line. When they cut the hog open on the line, the smell of the gangrene was so bad someone got sick. And those fellows have tough stomachs too. The farmer didn't get his money and was hopping mad. I had to go out and explain to him how the nerve damage was related to the gangrene."

The hog carcasses, as they leave the area for the cooler, are shining pink-white. Dr. Smith examines a side as it moves by him on the rail and has a small red bruise cut from the shoulder.

In the company cafeteria at noon, there are polite but distinct groups that form. The workers, in hard hats and aprons, sit together. The management and office employees congregate in another area. Dr. McDonnell and his inspectors assemble in a third area.

"The policy is not to encourage relationships with company employees," Dr. McDonnell says, adding cold water to his coffee. "This is a delicate issue, but the dangers are obvious. It could be something as simple as relaxing standards for a friend on the rail to accepting actual bribes. We've never had a problem with bribery here, but we follow the policy anyway.

"The watchdog for us, I guess, would be the Compliance and Evaluation section of the U.S.D.A.," Dr. McDonnell goes on. "Those people go into the stores and buy different products to check on quality and labeling. Compliance and evaluation is also concerned with illegal transportation of products."

After lunch the inspectors return to their posts. Don Engley, a lay food inspector, has been at Gorham for thirteen years. He works on the floor below the kill known as "offal." From the kill, stainless-steel chutes deliver various by-products of the hog for processing or delivery to tankage. Intestines are washed out for sausage casings. Specialty items, such as chitterlings, pigs' ears and feet are cleaned and packaged.

"We look for violations of cleanliness, both in the employees and in the meat. We also have to inspect packaging. We make sure that the packages have what the label says they have. The inspection legend and number has to be there too. We have almost no contact with employees. If I see something going on, I speak to the foreman, not to the workers directly. It's best to avoid any direct conflicts.

"The people who work here are union people. Their wages are very good and their benefits are better than ours. But there is more security in the inspection work, even if the starting pay is lower— at least once you get through the first training year."

Another inspector, Marcia Dios, covers one of the upstairs areas which handles the processing of meats. She is a processing inspector.

"We keep it pretty cool in here," Marcia says as she opens a sliding door and pulls it shut behind her. She glances quickly at the wall thermometer in the refrigerated room. The noise here comes from the machines mixing vats of spice and meats for cold cuts and hot dogs. Some of the mixtures are flecked with green olives, others are tinted red.

"It's all pretty much the same stuff," Marcia says. "Just different spices and combinations of meat. What we check for is largely labeling . . . making sure the inspection station legends and number are visible. These products are sent all over the country under different labels."

Passing through another set of doors, and through a long corridor, Marcia enters the intense heat of the canned ham cooking room. The canned hams are boiling on racks in large vats. A young company employee sits at one end of the room near a row of clocks, reading a book.

"Each vat has its own clock," Marcia says. "The hams have to be cooked according to a schedule. It depends on the size and whether the hams are to be refrigerated or kept in a cupboard."

In another room, hams are sent to be pumped with brine before they are smoked. The hams move along a stainless-steel conveyor belt and through a machine which plunges needles into the meat, injecting the brine.

"Inspectors come through on an irregular schedule," Marcia says. "If things are going well, I might come through once an hour. If there's a new foreman, or the machines have been acting up I'll come more often. What we are checking here is that the amount of salt brine put in the hams doesn't exceed the legal limits. The brine contains nitrates, salt, phosphates, ascorbic acids—all things we want to control." She takes a slide rule from her lab coat. The man working the machine pulls a ham from the line and places it on the scale. Then he sends it through the pumper and puts it back on the scale, reading the gain in weight out to Marcia. Marcia makes some calculations on the slide rule and some notes in her book.

In another room, vats of hams are soaking in brine. Two stainless-steel tubs have red condemned tags on them. The tubs are filled with odds and ends of sliced bacon.

"Spoiled," Marcia says, wrinkling her nose. "You could smell it." In the area where the bacons and hams come out of the smoke house, Marcia stops quickly and asks an employee to pick up a roll of Canadian bacon that has fallen off a rack. The employee does so, rinsing the plastic wrapping off first in water.

"The floors here are always greasy," Marcia says. "But in places where it's also hot, it gets really dangerous. It's one of the safety hazards. There is a regular schedule of scrub downs, but it builds up awfully fast. Actually, most of the injuries here are from knife cuts. People who work in packing houses traditionally have a high incidence of brucellosis. That's a disease people can get from hogs and cattle. People with active bruccelosis can run fevers, have headaches, sweating and anemia. It's not nearly as common now as it used to be. Overall, I have no hesitation about buying products that are made here. I think they are really clean, quality products."

Dr. Beeman, another inspector, is the veterinarian on the cattle and sheep kill. The killing and cleaning of the carcasses are done on one floor at Gorham. The sheep are done in a corner of the hangar-like room.

"The sheep are led in by what we call a Judas goat," Dr. Beeman explains. "The goat leads them up from the livestock pens. He knows where to get out, but the sheep don't." The sheep are stunned much as the hogs are. The noise here is even louder than in the hog kill. Some of the employees and inspectors wear special ear muffs to protect their hearing. The huge beef carcasses swing along on the same kind of rail as the hogs do, never touching each other. The men who shoot the cattle to stun them stand on a high platform above the animals.

"This can be dangerous. An animal can get loose occasionally," Dr. Beeman says.

The floors are covered with bits of trimmings and blood, despite the constant sweeping of the men in raincoats. The cattle carcasses are divided in halves by sawing down the back bone. The saws are dipped often into a sterilizer of 180° water.

"That's to insure against contamination of the meat, in case the saw should hit an abcess or something. Essentially, we have the same kind of inspection personnel here as on the hog kill—head inspectors, viscera, rail—with me doing the final determination."

Back in the U.S.D.A. office Dr. McDonnell is going over the design of a label with a colleague, to make sure the information is displayed properly.

"There are plenty of problems in this job," he says, shaking his head. "There are so many regulations. But basically, there are reasons behind them and a really critical job to be done. Even today you hear stories about food processing plants and how unwholesome the food is. That's not true here. I guess that's what can get to you—the feeling that you're getting it from both ends. The company thinks we're over-inspecting, the consumer thinks we aren't doing enough.

"I wish I could get out and talk to consumer groups. Our job has to do with consumer interests—to assure the consumer a safe, wholesome product from a sanitary facility. We're really part of the everyday life of the consumer—I think they should know about our work."

It is late afternoon. From his window, Dr. McDonnell can see the refrigerated semis being loaded with Gorham processed meats. A U.S.D.A. inspector is there on the docks, clipboard in hand.

"See how closely we watch things?" Dr. McDonnell says. "I'm really proud of that."

SUMMARY

DUTIES: *Inspectors are employed by federal and state agencies to inspect meat, poultry and products made from them. They are hired to insure that these products are wholesome and safe. They work on-site in slaughtering and processing plants under the supervision of a veterinarian. In addition to inspecting the products themselves, the meat and poultry inspectors examine packages for proper labeling.*

TRAINING: *A person must pass an exam on specialized knowledge obtained in the meat and poultry inspector training program. Entry into this program is based on civil service tests, experience with animals and the current need for new inspectors. A high-school education is helpful but not an absolute requirement. For more information, contact local state civil service agencies or:*

> *The Interagency Board of the U.S. Civil Service*
> *Examiners for Washington, D.C.*
> *1900 E Street NW*
> *Washington, D.C. 20415*

SALARY: *$9,000–11,000 to start. Experienced inspectors make over $14,000.*

RELATED OCCUPATIONS

SANITARIAN

DUTIES: *Works for local health departments. Inspects restaurants, swimming pools and other facilities for potential health hazards. Assists in solving health problems by cooperating with other public health officials and the community. Acts as a consultant to facilities that have potential health problems.*

TRAINING: *Most individuals employed in such positions have at least an undergraduate degree with some background in the biological sciences. Some have gone on to get a master's degree from a school of public health. For information about such programs, contact:*

> *National Environmental Health Association*
> *1600 Pennsylvania*
> *Denver, Colorado   80203*
>
> *or*
>
> *American Public Health Association*
> *1015 18th Street NW*
> *Washington, D.C.   20036*

SALARY: *$10,000–30,000 depending on location, experience and supervisory responsibilities.*

NEIGHBORHOOD HEALTH WORKER

DUTIES: *Works for neighborhood health centers and local health departments. Assists in rat control, lead poisoning programs in the community and door-to-door health education and disease screening programs.*

TRAINING: *Agencies prefer people from the community. No formal educational requirements. Contact local health departments about programs and employment opportunities.*

SALARY: *$6,000–12,000 depending on location and experience of the individual.*

HEALTH INSPECTOR

DUTIES: *Responsible for inspecting and licensing health facilities and investigating industrial work settings for compliance with health and safety standards. Responsible for enforcing federal, state and local health regulations. Acts as a consultant to a facility that is trying to comply with health and safety standards.*

TRAINING: *An undergraduate degree, with special training in the field, is usually required. Inservice education trains the individual for the particular duties involved. Contact local or state health departments for more information.*

SALARY: *$10,000–30,000 depending on training, experience and supervisory responsibilities.*

COMMUNITY HEALTH INVESTIGATOR

DUTIES: *Locates sources of disease in the community. May be a generalist or specialize in such areas as lead poisoning or venereal disease. Collects information about a health problem and explores leads. Assists in getting various groups and agencies to work effectively once source of problem has been identified.*

TRAINING: *Most investigators have an undergraduate degree. A background in biological science is not required. Some agencies prefer liberal-arts majors, since the job often requires adept diplomacy rather than scientific skills.*

SALARY: *$12,000–30,000 depending on location, experience and responsibilities.*

MEDICAL EPIDEMIOLOGIST

DUTIES: *"Chief detective" for disease control investigations. Assembles the evidence, tests out leads and plans strategy for dealing with a disease problem once it is identified. May work nationally for the Center for Disease Control or for state or local health departments. The job often involves the same pressure and drama of criminal investigations.*

TRAINING: *MD degree with some advanced training in epidemiology or public health. For more information, contact:*

American Public Health Association
1015 18th Street NW
Washington, D.C. 20036

SALARY: *$30,000–80,000 depending on location, experience and supervisory responsibilities.*

RESEARCHER-STATISTICIAN

DUTIES: *Responsible for part of a network that collects information on illness and diseases across the country. May work for a local health department, state health department or the National Center for Health Statistics. Information includes local statistics on births, deaths and hospitalizations, and this information is used to monitor health problems and assist in the identification of health hazards.*

TRAINING: *Varies. In smaller local health departments, the job is essentially a clerical one. Larger local health departments or state health departments employ individuals with specialized graduate training in biostatistics. Additional information about such programs can be obtained from:*

American Public Health Association
1015 18th Street NW
Washington, D.C. 20036

SALARY: *$15,000–30,000 depending on experience and responsibilities.*

VIROLOGIST/BACTERIOLOGIST

DUTIES: *Performs laboratory work to identify disease-causing viruses or bacteria. Develops vaccines for immunization programs and assists in the evaluation of their safety and effectiveness. Works for Center for Disease Control, drug manufacturers, or medical schools.*

TRAINING: *Ph.D in microbiology or virology. Strong undergraduate science background needed for admission to doctoral programs. Some obtain MD degree prior to doing their doctoral work. Doctoral programs in microbiology and virology exist in many of the larger medical schools.*

SALARY: *$30,000–60,000 depending on location, experience and responsibilities.*

PUBLIC HEALTH NURSE

DUTIES: *Participates in public health screening and immunization programs. Often involved in home care and maternal and child health programs. Works for local health departments, state health departments, federal health programs and voluntary agencies.*

TRAINING: *A RN degree and state licensure. Many obtain specialized Masters of Public Health degrees from a school of public health. For more information, contact:*

> *American Public Health Association*
> *1015 18th Street NW*
> *Washington, D.C. 20036*

SALARY: *$12,000–25,000 depending on location, experience and responsibilities.*

DENTAL HYGIENIST

DUTIES: *Provides preventive dental services under the supervision of a dentist. May work for school systems, public agencies or in a private dental practice. Duties include providing dental health education, screening for dental health problems, cleaning teeth and taking and developing dental X rays.*

TRAINING: *In order to become licensed a candidate must graduate from an accredited school of dental hygiene and pass a written and clinical examination. Applicants to such programs should be high-school graduates. Programs offer either three-year associate or four-year bachelor's degrees. The associate degree is sufficient for those who wish to work in a private dentist's office but the bachelor's degree is usually required for those who teach, do research and work in public or school health programs.*

SALARY: *$12,900 is the average salary.*

17

YOUR FUTURE IN HEALTH CARE

The people introduced in this book represent only a few of the 600 job titles in the health area. It is a complex, rapidly changing field and it faces serious problems. This chapter will try to give you some perspective on the problems and how they may affect work environments. Then, it will give some suggestions for approaching a health career.

CONFLICTS WITHIN THE HEALTH-CARE "TEAM"

In this century there have been drastic changes in the way health care is organized. In 1900, 60 percent of all health workers were physicians. Now, physicians represent only 8 percent of the health-care work force. The rest of the work force is made up of nonphysician health workers.

With this change in the composition of the work force has come talk about the "team" approach in health care. However, talking about a team approach and having one are two different things. The attitudes of health professionals don't change overnight. A team implies a sense of common purpose and a willingness to use the skills and abilities of each member. That hasn't happened as much in health care as many would like.

Look at the health-care occupational pyramid represented in Figure 1. The higher up you are on the pyramid the more extended and specialized your education, the greater your independence, the higher your status and the greater influence you are likely to have.

YOUR FUTURE IN HEALTH CARE 221

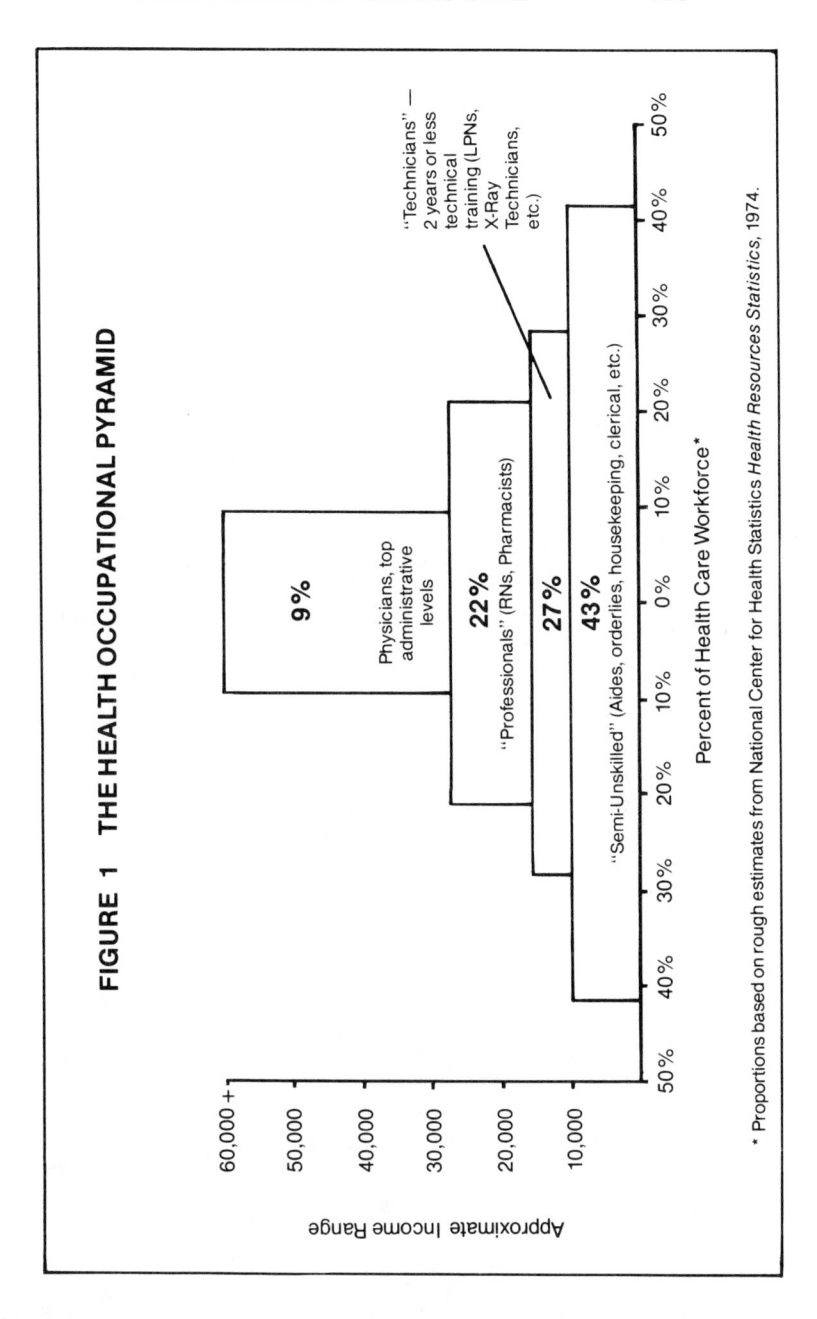

FIGURE 1 THE HEALTH OCCUPATIONAL PYRAMID

Approximate Income Range	Percent of Health Care Workforce*	Category
60,000+	9%	Physicians, top administrative levels
20,000–30,000	22%	"Professionals" (RNs, Pharmacists)
~15,000	27%	"Technicians"—2 years or less technical training (LPNs, X-Ray Technicians, etc.)
<10,000	43%	"Semi-Unskilled" (Aides, orderlies, housekeeping, clerical, etc.)

* Proportions based on rough estimates from National Center for Health Statistics *Health Resources Statistics*, 1974.

At the top of the pyramid are the physicians. They have achieved the highest degree of professional independence and status of any occupational group in the United States. At the bottom of the pyramid are nurses' aides and orderlies. They have been, at least until recently, poorly paid and given little if any formal training. They have performed the more routine and/or what are viewed as disagreeable tasks within an institution. The members of health-care teams include all the layers of the pyramid. They are dependent on each other and intimately involved with one another through the lives of patients. They should work like a team.

Imagine a professional football team organized the way a health team is organized. You have a superstar quarterback who gets a quarter of a million a year, has a glamorous jet-set lifestyle, doesn't have to show up at regular practice sessions, and orders his teammates around as if they were his servants. He's a passing quarterback, so if the linemen do their job, he won't even get his pants dirty. The linemen, on the other hand, get all the bruises, no headlines and $3.95 an hour. After a while, the linemen start thinking, "Hey, why don't we let some guys through to hit him?"

Some of this kind of friction crops up on the health-care team as well. It is made worse by the fact that health-care occupations are not part of the same *career ladder*. No matter how many years a person may work as a nurse's aide, s/he will not become a nurse. A nurse cannot expect, even with hard work and long hours, to become a physician. In most other kinds of work, there is a system for moving up. In health-care settings, it is greatly limited.

Since nurses can't become physicians and aides can't become nurses, each group sets about to better its own position in the pyramid. Each group does this by trying to model its own behavior after the highest group, the physicians. They increase training requirements for their members far beyond what is needed. They try to pass off the more disagreeable, routine tasks to people below them and take the more interesting, technically sophisticated tasks for themselves. Note the following anecdote in this regard:

A frail elderly woman turns white, gags, makes a desperate effort to hold it all down and then vomits on the floor next to her bed. A physician who has been examining another patient in the four-bed hospital room steps out in the hall and signals the head nurse.

"You'd better get somebody to clean that up," he says as he leaves.

The nurse asks the nurse's aide in the next room to come clean it up.
"Oh no, that's not part of my job. Get somebody in housekeeping to do it," she says, making a face.
The housekeeping person down the hall is equally reluctant.
"I just washed those floors. You people are supposed to take care of the patients," she says.
The head nurse, muttering angrily to herself, gets down on her knees on the floor and mops it up with a towel.

Buck-passing such as this happens a lot. When the buck stops, the one holding it is usually grumbling.

Sexism

There is another kind of conflict simmering within the health-care team. Unlike the football team, it is coed. However, despite the fact that it is coed, women and men are not equal. Look at the following report:

There was a head-on collision between two cars. The bodies of a mother and her daughter were removed from the wreckage of one automobile. The mother was dead, but the daughter, although severely mangled, was still alive when she was rushed to a nearby hospital. The nurse in the emergency room took one look at the girl, screamed "My God! My daughter!" and fainted. In the same accident the bodies of a father and son were removed from the other automobile. The father had died instantly in the crash, but the son, who was still alive, was rushed to the same hospital. A nationally known surgeon was called to perform a delicate emergency operation on the boy. The surgeon stared at the boy, grimaced, and in a steely, emotionless voice said, "I can't operate. That's my son."
(D. Smith and A. Kaluzny, *The White Labyrinth,* McCutchan, Berkeley, 1975, p. 17.)

As the above excerpt suggests, one doesn't expect to see a male nurse or a female surgeon. Women don't often hold the top positions nor men the lower ones. In most cases, women hold the bottom positions of the pyramid. Even though they comprise 75 percent of the health-care work force, their numbers are underrepresented in top positions. To a large extent, the jobs that men and women have in health care reflect traditional views about sex roles. Women assume the dietary duties, the housekeeping duties and the mothering-nurturing roles that are associated with nursing.

They are also expected to be submissive and leave the major decisions to males. Men have traditionally been the doctors, dentists and administrators. Profound changes are taking place, however. Jobs are being defined less in keeping with these stereotypes and more in keeping with ability.

Racism

Black Americans, Hispanic Americans and American Indians are unquestionably underrepresented in the health-care team, especially in the upper parts of the pyramid. These groups often live in areas where health manpower is in great demand, yet not available. While one out of every 560 white Americans becomes a physician, it is only one in 3,800 among blacks. While 11 percent of the population was black in 1970, only 3.6 percent of the registered nurses in the country was black. Figures for Hispanic Americans and American Indians are not any better. Statistics show that their presence in the health professions is minimal at best. Schools, the government and other organizations are encouraging minority students to enter the health professions by providing special funds for their education. Some of these are listed in Appendix B.

Administering to Whom?

Unlike a football team, the health-care team has two quarterbacks. One is responsible to the institution. This is the administrator or the director of nursing, depending on the situation. The other is the patient's physician. The physician isn't employed by the institution, but s/he gives orders to its staff and expects them to be carried out. The physician has one patient and s/he wants to make sure s/he gets the best care possible. The institution has many patients and its administrators have to keep things running as smoothly as possible. Often a health-care worker is caught in the middle. The rules of the institution may say, "Process all laboratory tests in the order that they come in except for real emergencies." The physician says, "Get me this lab test right away. I have to get back to my office in ten minutes and I want to make sure things are OK with Mrs. Jones." These kinds of conflicts may be part of work in health.

Carving Up the Pie

On a football team, everybody has a position and knows what s/he is supposed to do. On the health-care team, many times people can't agree about who should be playing what position or even what the positions are. Many registered nurses would like to eliminate aides and licensed practical nurses from hospital floors and handle all responsibilities themselves. Some physicians question the usefulness of physician extenders, while others would like to see their roles expanded. Each group wants to carve out as much turf as possible for itself.

It is sometimes hard to see how the health-care team can work at all. It does work, although most would agree not as well as it could. The work is neither stable nor free from conflicts, but it provides a stimulating challenge.

CONFLICTS WITH PUBLIC EXPECTATIONS

Presidents, members of Congress and spokespersons for organized medicine have been talking for years about the "crisis" in medical care. The health-care system is not providing what they or the public have come to expect. These conflicts seem to center around the three issues of cost, effectiveness and fairness.

Cost

Health care should be provided at a reasonable cost. Unfortunately, it is getting more and more expensive. The average person works six weeks out of the year just to pay her or his family medical bills. General Motors executives now complain that they are spending more money on health insurance for their employees than they are for the steel that goes into the cars they build. Union officials complain about the cost of health insurance too. They are tired of collective bargaining for their members when only the doctors and hospitals benefit from it. Members of Congress are also unhappy when they see the cost of the Medicare program doubling every four years. On the average, over the past ten years, the costs of health care have risen more than twice as fast as prices in general.

What is happening? Many things at the same time. Health-care workers at the bottom of the pyramid have become unionized. Their wages have caught up with those in other sectors of the economy. People are also using more health care than before. As our population becomes older, more health care is being demanded. Perhaps half of the increase, however, has come from changes in the practice of medicine. New technology, such as that involved with cardiac-care units, new X-ray equipment such as CAT scanners and new kinds of health workers, such as cardiac nurse specialists, have contributed to the cost increase. People are beginning to ask the question, "How much and what kind of health care can we afford?"

Effectiveness

The public might not be so concerned about the cost of health care if they could see some results. However, we aren't living any longer today than we did in 1950, yet, we are spending four times as much for our health care. Part of the problem is that we spend money on the wrong things. Too much is spent on costly technology, and too little on prevention, on primary care, on making the environment more healthy or on just caring for people. Preventive techniques are pushed aside, for the most part. They are not as glamorous as open-heart surgery, but they do tend to extend one's life expectancy. They keep the body healthy while operations only repair. From this perspective, people such as home health aides and health educators are more effective than has been recognized in the past. Their skills are of inestimable value.

It would be unfortunate if, to keep costs from rising, areas such as preventive medicine were restricted. Health System Agencies and local health planning groups that have a majority of consumers on their boards may help prevent this from happening. In any event, the health sector must push hard if it wants to receive public support in areas like preventive medicine. It must prove to the public that these new techniques are effective.

Fairness

We have come to view health care as a right. The idea that the wealthy can purchase longer, healthier lives than others is not acceptable to most people. Yet, the right to health care is more of a promise than a reality. Many people can't afford the care they need and are discreetly turned away. As much as half the population does not have adequate health insurance coverage for a serious illness. Those that need it most are the least likely to get care. Those expectant mothers most likely to have problems delivering their babies are the ones least likely to get regular examinations during pregnancy. Those in poorer, rural areas are often old and sick, but they are the ones less likely to have access to primary care. All of these instances point up the fact that everyone should have some minimal right to health care. But, as of yet, that right has not been adequately assured.

HOW CAN YOU FIT IN?

We have come through a period when it was fashionable to be hang-loose about work. People today want jobs—not just jobs, but careers, work that provides a sense of identity and purpose beyond the security of a paycheck. Health occupations provide opportunities for a wide range of interests and educational aspirations. The future of the job market in the health areas seems secure. Pay scales and professional status are rising across the board. How do you approach the question of whether you belong and where you might fit in?

It is reasonable to ask a child, "What will you be when you grow up?" But for people who face concrete career decisions, the question can be a paralyzing one. Fortunately, it is not a matter of answering that one menacing question. Career development is a lifetime process. It comes with the answers to hundreds of smaller questions. It should be clear from reading about the careers of people in this book that getting into a health occupation is not a matter of making a single decision. There is a different route for every person. If you want it, there can be one for you.

Training

Competition to get into training programs in health occupations is increasing.

"We have a two-year wait in our nursing programs," reports a guidance counselor at a community college. "There are similar back-ups in other areas. The only exceptions would be medical technicians and dental technicians because they work in private offices and don't make as much money."

Planning in advance is clearly important. Identifying good programs, applying early and having alternatives should be your goals. Appendix A will provide you with a list of state organizations responsible for health occupations education. They should supply you with lists of available training programs in hospitals, vocational-technical schools, community colleges and four-year colleges. The professional organizations listed at the end of each chapter under "Related Occupations" can also be used for such information.

The pressure and competition in health training programs may come as a surprise to people who think of vocational courses as easy.

"This is part of the whole turn toward professionalism in the allied health occupations," a counselor reports. "The teachers are really concerned about not letting someone out to work who will screw up and bring a bad name to their program. They are uptight about the programs being accredited. Sometimes students who seem unstable or are having trouble keeping up are dealt with pretty heavy handedly. For students who have a hard time with the class work in a technical training program, we sometimes recommend a shorter, easier nurse's aide program and a job for a while to build up their confidence. Then they might be able to come back to the technical program."

Once in a training program, especially one that is difficult to get into, there is a tendency for students to get on the track and never look around. A health occupations adviser for a large university warned about this tendency.

"Health students get very uptight, very competitive during their training. Their problem is different from the four-year liberal-arts student, who hangs loose until the end of her or his senior year and then says 'My God! What am I going to do with a degree in Ancient History?' The health student is being trained for a specific job. The job market is excellent. Because of the specialized skills and the good job opportunities, students are really afraid to question whether they are doing the right thing. We recommend a periodic self-evaluation, just a pause to think. We are ready to point to alternatives if someone has second thoughts."

Training does not have to be seen in terms of a one-way ticket. While advancement in one health occupation does not bring standing in another, people can find ways to move. An operating room technician might choose to work for a registered nursing degree, or a two-year registered nurse might find a way to complete a bachelor's degree on the side. Gaining experience and confidence in one area can be an impetus to training in another area. This may take more of an effort in the health fields than it does in other fields, but it is done. There is also an effort in some training programs to give credit for experience in other branches of health work.

Financing Your Training

Financing training for health occupations is much the same as for other schooling. Few scholarships cover all expenses. Financial assistance will probably come from several sources—family loans, part-time work, scholarships and/or student loans from banks or the government. Information on financing is usually made available when you apply for a training program at a school. Appendix B gives a list of specific organizations involved with financial aid to health occupation students.

A Talk, a Letter and Get to Work

In venturing into the health field, remember that the first step is in many ways the hardest. Once you have started, one step tends to lead to another. With each step, the decision about the next one becomes clearer. We have listed some of the organizations to contact. Additional information is available from libraries, schools and counselors. For a start, we would suggest the following: a talk, a letter and getting to work.

A Talk. The talk should be with someone working in a health career that is of interest to you. With so many different health careers, meeting someone in your interest area is best not left to chance. Make an appointment with a family friend or a friend of a friend, or call a local hospital and track someone down. People like to talk about their work, and in health professions, particularly, there is a new pride and eagerness to let people know what is going on. Ask how they got into their work. Ask about your own fears, about training, about work-related problems. The information you get from health workers will improve your ability to make a decision.

Write a Letter. In addition to collecting your personal information on health work, get some materials about training programs from one of the organizations listed in Appendix A. Write directly to colleges and vocational schools for their course brochures and applications. When you begin to see the differences in the programs, your decisions may become easier.

Get to Work. Above all, try to do some work in a health-care setting. It may not be the kind of work you do after training, but getting involved will have three major benefits for you. It will give you a feel for the routine of caring for people. It will introduce you to other health occupations and give you a chance to talk to health workers. In addition, schools and employers will look at your work experiences as a sign of your seriousness about health work.

The kind of work you will be able to do will vary greatly depending on the needs in your area. In some places, work as nurses' aides and orderlies is readily available. In others, the competition is high. Call your area hospitals and inquire about job possibilities. If you are too young to work, or if there are no jobs available, ask about volunteer work at hospitals, nursing homes or special schools, such as those for retarded children. From a volunteer position, you might work your way into a job. If not, the experience will still be a valuable addition to your view of health work. Some high schools incorporate job experience into the final year or two of school. Find out if these programs are available in your area.

You must make the first move toward a health occupation. But if you take that first step, there is information and help available to set you on your way.

APPENDIX A: STATE OFFICIALS RESPONSIBLE FOR HEALTH OCCUPATIONS EDUCATION

State	Name and Title	Address
Alabama	State Supervisor Health Occupations Education	Division of Vocational Education State Department of Education Montgomery, Alabama 36130 (205) 832-5337
	Specialist Health Occupations Education	University of Alabama P.O. Box 2847 University, Alabama 34586 (205) 348-4576
Alaska	State Supervisor Health Occupations Education	Division of Vocational Education Pouch F Alaska Office Building Juneau, Alaska 99801 (907) 465-2980
Arizona	Specialist Health Occupations Education	Division of Career and Vocational Education 1535 West Jefferson Phoenix, Arizona 85007 (602) 271-5485
	Deputy Associate Superintendent for Program Services	address same as above (602) 271-5832
Arkansas	Director Health Occupations Education	State Department of Education Arch Ford Education Building Little Rock, Arkansas 72201 (501) 371-2361
California	Specialist Health Occupations	Occupational Education California Community College 1238 S Street, Room 204 Sacramento, California 95814 (916) 445-0486

State	Name and Title	Address
	Consultant Health Careers and Services	Bureau of Industrial Education 721 Capitol Mall Sacramento, California 95814 (916) 445-2461
Colorado	Supervisor Health Occupations Education	207 State Services Building Denver, Colorado 80203 (303) 892-3162
Connecticut	Consultant Health Occupations Education	State Department of Education State Office Building Room 343 Box 2219 Hartford, Connecticut 06115 (203) 566-4561
	Associate Consultant Health Occupations Education	State Office Building Room 344 Box 2219 Hartford, Connecticut 06115 (203) 566-7117
Delaware	State Supervisor Home Economics and Related Occupations	State Department of Public Instruction Box 697 Dover, Delaware 19901 (302) 678-4681
District of Columbia	Supervising Director Health Occupations Education	M. M. Washington Vocational Center 27 O Street, N.W. Washington, D.C. 20001 (202) 673-7224
Florida	Director Health and Public Service Education	Florida Department of Education Knott Building Tallahassee, Florida 32304 (904) 488-7431
	Consultant Health and Public Service Education	address and phone as above
	Consultant Health Occupations Student Organization	address and phone as above
Georgia	Director Health Occupations Education	340 State Office Building State Department of Education Atlanta, Georgia 30334 (404) 656-2550

APPENDIX A

State	Name and Title	Address
	Assistant Professor Health Occupations Education	The University of Georgia Division of Vocational Education 411 Tucker Hall Athens, Georgia 30601 (404) 542-8595
Guam	Associate Superintendent Career & Occupational Education	Division of Careers and Occupations Department of Education P.O. Box DE Agana, Guam 96910 9-0 Overseas 72-785
Hawaii	State Director for Vocational Education	University of Hawaii Bachman 101 2444 Dole Street Honolulu, Hawaii 96822 (808) 948-7461
Idaho	Assistant State Supervisor Trade and Industrial and Health Occupations Education	State Board for Vocational Education 650 West State Street Boise, Idaho 83720 (208) 384-3271
Illinois	Head Consultant Health Occupations Education	State Board of Education Illinois Office of Education 100 North First Street Springfield, Illinois 62777 (217) 782-4877
	Consultant Health Occupations Education	Address and phone same as above
	Consultant Health Occupations Education	Address and phone same as above
Indiana	Chief Consultant Health Occupations Education	Division of Vocational and Technical Education Department of Public Instruction 16th Floor 120 West Market Street Indianapolis, Indiana 46204 (317) 633-4841
Iowa	Senior State Consultant Health Occupations Education	135 Melrose Avenue Iowa City, Iowa 52240 (319) 353-3536

State	Name and Title	Address
Kansas	Education Program Specialist Health Occupations Education	State Department of Education 120 East Tenth Street Topeka, Kansas 66612 (913) 296-2227
Kentucky	Director Health and Personal Services Occupations Unit	Capitol Plaza Tower, 21st Floor Frankfort, Kentucky 40601 (502) 564-3775
Louisiana	State Supervisor Health Occupations Education	Capitol Station P.O. Box 44064 Baton Rouge, Louisiana 70804 (504) 389-2991
Maine	State Supervisor Health Occupations Education	State Department of Education State Office Building Augusta, Maine 04333 (207) 289-3565
Maryland	State Specialist Health Occupations Education	State Department of Education P.O. Box 8717 Baltimore-Washington International Airport Baltimore, Maryland 21240 (301) 796-8300
Massachusetts	Director Bureau of Program Services	Division of Occupational Education State Department of Education 31 St. James Avenue Boston, Massachusetts 02116 (617) 727-5730
	Coordinator Office of Private Schools	Address same as above (617) 727-5738
Michigan	Specialist Postsecondary Health Occupations Education	Vocational Technical Education Service P.O. Box 30009 Lansing, Michigan 48909 (517) 373-3360
Minnesota	Vocational Program Supervisor Postsecondary Health Occupations Education	State Department of Education 546 Capitol Square 550 Cedar Street St. Paul, Minnesota 55101 (612) 296-3755

State	Name and Title	Address
	Vocational Program Supervisor Secondary Health Occupations Education	State Department of Education 516 Capitol Square 550 Cedar Street St. Paul, Minnesota 55101 (612) 296-4864
	Vocational Program Supervisor Adult Health Occupations Education	State Department of Education 525 Capitol Square 550 Cedar Street St. Paul, Minnesota 55101 (612) 296-6516
Mississippi	State Supervisor Health Occupations Education	Division of Vocational Education State Department of Education Box 771 Jackson, Mississippi 39205 (601) 354-6860
Missouri	State Supervisor Health Occupations Education	State Department of Education P.O. Box 480 Jefferson City, Missouri 65101 (314) 751-4460
Montana	State Consultant Health Occupations Education	Office of Public Instruction State Capitol Helena, Montana 59601 (406) 449-2087
Nebraska	Director Trade and Industrial and Health Occupations Education	301 Centennial Mall South 6th Floor Box 94987 Lincoln, Nebraska 68509 (402) 471-2441
Nevada	Supervisor Health Occupations Education	State Department of Education Carson City, Nevada 89701 (702) 885-5700 Ext. 255
New Hampshire	Supervisor Health Occupations Education	State Department of Education Division of Vocational-Technical Education 105 Loudon Road—Prescott Park Concord, New Hampshire 03301 (603) 271-2662
New Jersey	Director Health Occupations Education	Division of Vocational Education State Department of Education 225 West State Street Trenton, New Jersey 08625 (609) 292-6592

State	Name and Title	Address
	Consultant Health Careers	Address same as above (609) 292-6593
New Mexico	State Supervisor Health Occupations Education	Division of Vocational Education State Department of Education Education Building Santa Fe, New Mexico 87503 (505) 827-3151
New York	Chief Bureau of Health Occupations Education	Division of Occupational Education Instruction Office of Occupational and Continuing Education State Education Department 99 Washington Avenue Albany, New York 12230 (518) 474-1711
North Carolina	Chief Consultant Health Occupations Education	State Department of Public Instruction Education Building Raleigh, North Carolina 27611 (919) 733-2519
North Dakota	Supervisor Trade, Technical, and Health Occupations	State Board for Vocational Education State Office Building 900 East Boulevard Bismarck, North Dakota 58505 (701) 224-3183
Ohio	State Supervisor Health Occupations Education	State Department of Education 65 South Front Street Room 914 Columbus, Ohio 43215 (614) 466-2901
Oklahoma	State Supervisor Health Occupations Education	State Department of Education Vocational-Technical Education 4024 Lincoln Boulevard Oklahoma City, Oklahoma 73105 (405) 521-3305
Oregon	Specialist Health Occupations Education	State Department of Education 942 Lancaster Drive, N.E. Salem, Oregon 97310 (503) 378-3590

APPENDIX A

State	Name and Title	Address
Pennsylvania	Senior Program Specialist Health Occupations Education	Department of Education Box 911 Harrisburg, Pennsylvania 17126 (717) 787-8862
Puerto Rico	Director Health Occupations Programs	Division of Vocational Education Department of Education P.O. Box 765 Hato Ray, Puerto Rico 00919 (809) 766-9010
	Program Coordinator Mayaquez Region	Eugenio M. de Hosto Vocational School Mayaquez, Puerto Rico 00708
Rhode Island	Coordinator	Bureau of Vocational-Technical Education Rhode Island Department of Education Roger Williams Building Room 301 Hayes Street Providence, Rhode Island 02908 (401) 277-2691
South Carolina	State Supervisor Health Occupations Education	Department of Vocational Education State Department of Education Rutledge Office Building Columbia, South Carolina 29201 (803) 758-2163
South Dakota	Supervisor Health Occupations Education and Special Needs Programs	Division of Vocational Education New Office Building Pierre, South Dakota 57501 (605) 224-3423
Tennessee	Head State Specialist Health Occupations Education	State Department of Education 208 Cordell Hull Building Nashville, Tennessee 37219 (615) 741-1931
Texas	Director Health Occupations Education Secondary Health Occupations	Department of Occupational Education and Technology Texas Education Agency 201 East 11th Street Austin, Texas 78701 (512) 475-4796

State	Name and Title	Address
Utah	State Specialist Health Occupations Education	250 East 5th South Salt Lake City, Utah 84111 (801) 533-5371
Vermont	Consultant Health Occupations Education	State Department of Education State Office Building Montpelier, Vermont 05602 (802) 828-3101
Virginia	Supervisor Health Occupations Education	P.O. Box 6 Q State Department of Education State Office Building Richmond, Virginia 23216 (804) 786-7110
Virgin Islands	State Director Vocational-Technical Education	Department of Education St. Thomas, Virgin Islands 00801 (809) 774-3046
Washington	Program Supervisor Health Occupations Education	Vocational Education State Superintendent of Public Instruction Old Capitol Building Olympia, Washington 98504 (206) 753-5650
West Virginia	State Supervisor Health Occupations Education	1900 Washington Street East Room B-237 Charleston, West Virginia 25305 (304) 348-2389
Wisconsin	Consultant Health Occupations Education	Wisconsin Board of Vocational, Technical, and Adult Education Hill Farms State Office Building 7th Floor 4802 Sheboygan Avenue Madison, Wisconsin 53702 (608) 266-0003
Wyoming	Coordinator Distributive Education and Health Occupations Education	State Department of Education Hathaway Building Cheyenne, Wyoming 82002 (307) 777-7411

APPENDIX B: INFORMATION ON FINANCIAL AID

The following is a list of publications and organizations where you might get information on financial aid.

College Costs Today, New York Life Insurance Company, Free. Available from any New York Life agent.

Health Careers Guidebook, 3rd Edition, Superintendent of Documents, U.S. Government Printing Office, Washington, D.C. 20402. Stock Number 2900-0158, $2.25.

Health Professions Student Loan Program, Bureau of Health Resources Development, Health Resources Administration, U.S. Department of Health Education and Welfare, 9000 Rockville Pike, Bethesda, Maryland 20014. Free.

How Medical Students Finance Their Education, Bureau of Health Resources Development, Health Resources Administration, Department of Health Education and Welfare, 9000 Rockville Pike, Bethesda, Maryland 20014. Free.

Join the Life Corps (same as above).

Need a Lift? (information on careers, loans, scholarships, and student employment) American Legion Educational and Scholarship Program, American Legion, Dept. S, PO Box 1055, Indianapolis, Indiana 46206. 50¢.

Nursing Student Loan Program, Bureau of Health Resources Development, Health Resources Administration, Department of Health Education and Welfare, 9000 Rockville Pike, Bethesda, Maryland 20014. Free.

Scholarships for American Indians, Bureau of Indian Affairs Higher Education Program, PO Box 1788, Albuquerque, New Mexico 87103. Free.

Where to Get Health Career Information, National Health Council, 1740 Broadway, New York, New York 10019. Free.